THE CANCER SOLUTION : PROVEN METHODS TO CONTROL AND COMBAT THE DISEASE

THE CANCER SOLUTION : PROVEN METHODS TO CONTROL AND COMBAT THE DISEASE

Table of Contents

INTRODUCTION

The Cancer Solution: Proven Methods to Control and Combat the Disease."In a world where cancer affects millions of lives each year, this book seeks to empower you with knowledge and strategies to face this formidable adversary head-on. Through extensive research, expert insights, and real-life experiences, we have crafted a comprehensive guide to help you understand the complexities of cancer, its causes, and most importantly, the proven methods to prevent, control, and combat it.
Cancer is a disease that knows no boundaries, affecting individuals of all ages, backgrounds, and walks of life. Its impact extends beyond the patient, encompassing their families, friends, and communities. With such far-reaching consequences, it becomes crucial to equip ourselves with the right tools to address this challenge effectively.
Throughout the pages of this book, you will delve into the foundations of cancer prevention, exploring the vital role lifestyle factors play in reducing risks. We will dive into the importance of early detection and diagnosis, discussing the latest advancements in diagnostic tools that enhance our ability to catch cancer at its earliest stages.
While conventional cancer treatments have been the standard for many years, we will also explore complementary and alternative therapies that can augment traditional approaches. Integrative cancer care, which seeks to combine the best of both worlds, will be thoroughly examined to aid in creating personalized treatment plans tailored to individual needs.
Moreover, this book will bring you up-to-date on the most promising advances in cancer research, such as

immunotherapy and targeted therapies, providing hope for a future where cancer can be effectively managed and controlled.

Cancer survivorship and support will be discussed in detail, focusing on ways to cope with life after cancer and nurture physical and emotional well-being. Additionally, we will delve into strategies to prevent cancer recurrence and ways to empower yourself and your loved ones on this journey.

"The Cancer Solution"is not just a book; it is a source of empowerment and inspiration. By the time you reach the last page, we hope you will feel equipped to face cancer with confidence and determination. Let us embark on this journey together, arming ourselves with knowledge and proven methods to control and combat this disease, and ultimately, to envision a cancer-free future.

Chapter 1

Understanding Cancer: Causes and Prevalence

Cancer is a leading cause of morbidity and mortality globally. The exact causes of cancer can be attributed to a combination of genetic, environmental, and lifestyle factors. Genetic mutations can arise spontaneously or be inherited, increasing the risk of certain cancers. Environmental factors, such as exposure to radiation, chemicals, and pollutants, can also contribute to the development of cancer. Additionally, lifestyle choices like tobacco and alcohol use, poor diet, lack of physical activity, and excessive sun exposure have been linked to an increased risk of various cancers.

The prevalence of cancer varies across different populations and regions. Age is a significant factor, as the risk of developing cancer tends to increase with age. Certain types of cancer are more common in specific demographics. For instance, breast cancer is prevalent among women, while prostate cancer is more frequently diagnosed in men. Geographical factors also play a role, with variations in cancer prevalence attributed to differences in lifestyle, environmental exposures, and access to healthcare.

Early detection and advances in medical technology have improved cancer outcomes. Screening tests, such as mammograms and colonoscopies, enable the identification of cancer at an earlier, more treatable stage. Cancer treatment options include surgery, chemotherapy, radiation therapy, immunotherapy, and targeted therapy. Personalized medicine, which tailors treatment plans based on an individual's genetic makeup, is an emerging approach that holds promise for more effective and precise cancer treatment.

Raising awareness about cancer prevention is crucial in reducing its prevalence. Public health campaigns advocate for healthy lifestyle choices, including maintaining a balanced diet, engaging in regular physical activity, avoiding tobacco and excessive alcohol consumption, and using sun protection. Understanding the causes and prevalence of cancer empowers individuals to make informed decisions about their health and take proactive steps towards prevention and early detection.

1.1 The Need for Effective Cancer Control and Combat

Cancer continues to be a significant global health challenge, affecting millions of lives and causing considerable socio-economic burdens. The urgency for effective cancer control and combat is evident as the disease's prevalence continues to rise and impact individuals, families, and healthcare systems around the world.

1. Escalating Cancer Cases: The incidence of cancer is escalating due to factors such as population growth, aging, and lifestyle changes. As populations expand and age, the number of cancer cases is projected to increase, posing a considerable strain on healthcare infrastructure, resources, and services.

2. Humanitarian Impact: The impact of cancer extends beyond physical health, affecting emotional well-being, financial stability, and overall quality of life. Families and caregivers often bear the emotional and financial burdens of cancer treatment, which can lead to reduced productivity, increased poverty, and compromised social welfare.

3. Healthcare Systems: The burden on healthcare systems is immense. Cancer diagnosis, treatment, and management require specialized medical expertise, advanced technology, and a range of supportive services. Overwhelmed healthcare systems may struggle to provide timely and adequate care, leading to disparities in access to treatment and poorer outcomes.

4. Economic Considerations: The economic impact of cancer is substantial. Direct medical costs, including treatments, hospitalizations, and follow-up care, can be financially crippling. Indirect costs, such as lost productivity and premature death, further exacerbate the economic burden on societies.

5. Prevention and Early Detection: Effective cancer control strategies emphasize prevention and early detection. Encouraging healthy lifestyles, promoting awareness of risk factors, and implementing regular screenings can lead to the identification of cancer at earlier stages, when treatment is often more successful and less invasive.

6. Research and Innovation: Advances in research and medical technology play a vital role in combating cancer. Funding and support for cancer research drive the development of new therapies, targeted treatments, and innovative diagnostic tools, offering hope for improved outcomes and enhanced patient care.

7. Global Collaboration: Cancer knows no boundaries, making international collaboration essential. Sharing knowledge, expertise, and resources across countries and regions can accelerate progress in cancer control. Collaborative efforts can help bridge gaps in access to treatment, reduce disparities, and promote best practices.

8. Patient-Centered Care: An effective cancer control approach places patients at the center. Providing holistic care that addresses physical, emotional, and psychosocial needs is crucial for improving the overall well-being of individuals diagnosed with cancer and their families.

Chapter 2

Foundation of Cancer Control

Cancer control is built upon a multifaceted foundation encompassing various strategies aimed at preventing, detecting, treating, and managing cancer. This comprehensive approach involves collaboration between healthcare systems, governments, organizations, researchers, and communities to address the challenges posed by cancer and improve public health outcomes. The foundation of cancer control is grounded in several key pillars:

1. Prevention and Risk Reduction: The cornerstone of cancer control is prevention. Efforts to reduce cancer risk involve raising awareness about lifestyle factors such as tobacco and alcohol use, maintaining a healthy diet, engaging in regular physical activity, and practicing sun safety. Vaccination against certain cancer-causing viruses, such as HPV, also plays a pivotal role in prevention.

2. Early Detection and Screening: Timely detection can significantly improve cancer outcomes. Cancer screening programs, which include tests like mammograms, Pap smears, and colonoscopies, enable the identification of cancer at an early, more treatable stage. Effective communication and education about the importance of screening are essential components of this pillar.

3. Quality Treatment and Care: Providing access to quality cancer treatment and care is paramount. Healthcare systems must ensure that cancer patients have access to appropriate medical facilities, skilled healthcare professionals, and state-of-the-art treatments. Equitable access to treatment helps mitigate disparities in outcomes.

4. Research and Innovation: Cancer control relies on continuous research and innovation. Scientists and researchers strive to uncover new insights into cancer biology, develop targeted therapies, and enhance diagnostic tools. Funding and support for cancer research drive progress toward improved treatments and personalized medicine.

5. Global Collaboration: International cooperation is vital in addressing the global burden of cancer. Collaborative efforts enable the sharing of best practices, resources, and expertise across borders. Global partnerships can accelerate progress in cancer control and facilitate the exchange of knowledge and innovations.

6. Public Awareness and Education: Raising public awareness about cancer, its risk factors, and available resources is crucial. Educational campaigns empower individuals to make informed decisions about their health and encourage early detection and healthy behaviors.

7. Policy and Advocacy: Government policies and advocacy initiatives play a pivotal role in shaping cancer control efforts. Implementing regulations related to tobacco control, promoting healthy environments, and allocating resources for cancer research and healthcare services are essential steps in combating cancer.

8. Patient Empowerment: Empowering cancer patients and survivors is central to effective cancer control. Providing psychosocial support, patient-centered care, and survivorship programs helps individuals navigate the challenges of cancer and improve their overall quality of life.

9. Monitoring and Evaluation: Regular monitoring and evaluation of cancer control programs allow for the assessment of their effectiveness. Data collection and analysis help identify areas for improvement, guide resource allocation, and ensure that cancer control efforts remain evidence-based and impactful.

2.1 Lifestyle Factors and Their Impact on Cancer

Lifestyle choices play a significant role in influencing an individual's risk of developing cancer. These modifiable factors can either contribute to or mitigate the likelihood of cancer occurrence. Understanding the relationship between lifestyle choices and cancer risk is crucial for promoting prevention and overall well-being. Several key lifestyle factors and their impact on cancer are outlined below:

1. Tobacco Use: Smoking is one of the most well-established risk factors for cancer. It is linked to various types of cancer, including lung, mouth, throat, esophagus, pancreas, bladder, and kidney cancers. Secondhand smoke exposure is also associated with an increased risk. Quitting smoking or avoiding tobacco use altogether significantly reduces the risk of developing these cancers.

2. Alcohol Consumption: Excessive alcohol consumption is associated with an increased risk of several cancers, such as mouth, throat, esophagus, liver, breast, and colorectal cancers. Limiting alcohol intake and adhering to recommended guidelines can help lower the risk of these cancers.

3. Diet and Nutrition: A diet high in fruits, vegetables, whole grains, and lean proteins is linked to a reduced risk of cancer. On the other hand, diets high in processed meats, red meats, sugary foods, and excessive calories are associated with an increased risk of colorectal, stomach, and other cancers. A balanced and nutritious diet can contribute to overall health and lower cancer risk.

4. Physical Activity: Regular physical activity has a protective effect against cancer. Engaging in moderate to vigorous exercise helps maintain a healthy weight, reduce inflammation, and improve immune function. It is associated with a lower risk of breast, colon, and endometrial cancers.

5. Body Weight: Maintaining a healthy body weight is essential for cancer prevention. Obesity is linked to an increased risk of several cancers, including breast, colorectal, pancreatic, and kidney cancers. Achieving and maintaining a healthy weight through diet and exercise is a key strategy for reducing cancer risk.

6. Sun Exposure: Overexposure to ultraviolet (UV) radiation from the sun or tanning beds is a major risk factor for skin cancer, including melanoma, the deadliest form of skin cancer. Protecting the skin with sunscreen, clothing, and seeking shade can help prevent skin cancer.

7. Infections: Infections with certain viruses and bacteria can increase the risk of developing cancer. For example, chronic infection with hepatitis B or C viruses is associated with liver cancer, and human papillomavirus (HPV) infection is a leading cause of cervical and other cancers. Vaccination and safe practices can reduce the risk of these infections and associated cancers.

8. Environmental Exposures: Exposure to environmental pollutants, such as asbestos, radon, and certain chemicals, can contribute to cancer risk. Minimizing exposure to these substances in workplaces and living environments is important for prevention.

2.2 Diet and Nutrition for Cancer Prevention

A well-balanced and nutrient-rich diet plays a vital role in reducing the risk of cancer. The foods we consume can influence various biological processes, including inflammation, oxidative stress, and hormone regulation, all of which are linked to cancer development. By making mindful dietary choices, individuals can take proactive steps toward preventing cancer. Here are key principles for incorporating diet and nutrition into a cancer prevention strategy:

1. Plant-Based Foods: Emphasize a diet rich in fruits, vegetables, whole grains, legumes, nuts, and seeds. These plant-based foods are high in vitamins, minerals, fiber, and antioxidants, which help protect cells from damage and support overall health.

2. Colorful Variety: Consume a wide range of colorful fruits and vegetables. Different colors often indicate different types of antioxidants and phytochemicals, which have diverse protective properties. Aim to "eat the rainbow"to maximize nutrient intake.

3. Lean Proteins: Choose lean protein sources such as poultry, fish, beans, lentils, and tofu. Minimize consumption of processed and red meats, as their link to certain cancers, particularly colorectal cancer, has been well-documented.

4. Whole Grains: Opt for whole grains like brown rice, quinoa, whole wheat, and oats. These grains are rich in fiber and nutrients that contribute to a healthy digestive system and can help prevent colorectal cancer.

5. Healthy Fats: Include sources of healthy fats, such as avocados, nuts, seeds, and olive oil. Omega-3 fatty acids found in fatty fish like salmon also have anti-inflammatory properties and may contribute to cancer prevention.

6. Limit Sugars and Refined Carbohydrates: Minimize consumption of sugary foods and beverages, as well as foods high in refined carbohydrates. High sugar intake and rapid spikes in blood sugar levels have been associated with an increased risk of certain cancers.

7. Portion Control: Practice portion control to maintain a healthy weight. Excess body weight is a significant risk factor for various cancers, so controlling portion sizes can help prevent overeating and weight gain.

8. Hydration: Stay well-hydrated by drinking plenty of water. Adequate hydration supports proper bodily functions and helps maintain a healthy weight.

9. Moderate Alcohol Consumption: If you choose to consume alcohol, do so in moderation. Excessive alcohol intake is associated with an increased risk of certain cancers, including breast, liver, and esophageal cancers.

10. Limit Processed and Fast Foods: Minimize the consumption of processed and fast foods, which are often high in unhealthy fats, salt, and added sugars. These foods contribute to poor health and an increased risk of cancer.

11. Cooking Methods: Opt for healthier cooking methods such as steaming, grilling, baking, or sautéing, rather than deep-frying or charring foods, which can produce potentially harmful compounds.

12. Stay Informed: Keep up-to-date with nutritional guidelines and recommendations from reputable health organizations. Consulting with a registered dietitian can provide personalized guidance tailored to your individual health needs.

While no single food or nutrient can guarantee cancer prevention, adopting a balanced and healthful diet as part of an overall healthy lifestyle can significantly contribute to reducing cancer risk. Making thoughtful dietary choices can empower individuals to take control of their health and well-being, promoting a lifelong journey of cancer prevention.

2.3 Exercise and Physical Activity in Cancer Risk Reduction

Engaging in regular exercise and maintaining an active lifestyle are powerful strategies for reducing the risk of cancer. Physical activity not only contributes to overall well-being but also influences numerous biological processes that can help prevent the development of cancer. Incorporating exercise into daily routines can have a profound impact on health and play a significant role in cancer risk reduction. Here's how exercise contributes to cancer prevention:

1. Maintaining a Healthy Weight: Regular physical activity helps control body weight by burning calories and increasing metabolism. Maintaining a healthy weight is crucial, as obesity is a known risk factor for various types of cancer, including breast, colorectal, endometrial, and kidney cancers.

2. Reducing Inflammation: Exercise has anti-inflammatory effects on the body, which can help mitigate chronic inflammation a process associated with cancer development. By lowering inflammation, physical activity contributes to a healthier environment for cell growth and function.

3. Enhancing Immune Function: Physical activity supports a strong immune system, which plays a vital role in identifying and eliminating abnormal cells that can lead to cancer. Regular exercise improves immune response and surveillance, potentially reducing the risk of cancer.

4. Improving Hormone Regulation: Hormone levels play a significant role in cancer development. Physical activity can help regulate hormones such as insulin and estrogen, reducing the risk of hormone-related cancers like breast and endometrial cancer.

5. Promoting Digestive Health: Physical activity supports a healthy digestive system and regular bowel movements, reducing the time that potentially harmful substances remain in the colon. This can contribute to a lower risk of colorectal cancer.

6. Enhancing Oxygen Delivery: Exercise improves cardiovascular health and enhances oxygen delivery to tissues. This oxygenation helps maintain healthy cell function and can reduce the risk of certain cancers that thrive in low-oxygen environments.

7. Managing Blood Sugar Levels: Regular exercise improves insulin sensitivity and helps manage blood sugar levels. Elevated blood sugar levels are associated with an increased risk of certain cancers, so controlling blood sugar through physical activity can contribute to prevention.

8. Stress Reduction: Physical activity is a natural stress reliever and can have positive effects on mental well-being. Reducing chronic stress may indirectly contribute to cancer risk reduction by promoting a healthier physiological environment.

9. Healthy Aging: Regular exercise contributes to healthy aging by maintaining muscle mass, bone density, and cognitive function. It can also help prevent chronic conditions associated with aging, which can indirectly impact cancer risk.

10. Types of Exercise: Both aerobic exercises (e.g., walking, jogging, swimming) and strength training (e.g., weight lifting, resistance exercises) offer unique benefits. A combination of these exercises provides a comprehensive approach to overall health and cancer prevention.

It's important to note that any amount of physical activity is beneficial. Even small increases in daily movement can contribute to improved health and reduced cancer risk. Consult with a healthcare professional before starting a new exercise routine, especially if you have pre-existing health conditions.

Chapter 3

Early Detection and Diagnosis

Early detection and diagnosis are critical components of effective cancer management and treatment. Detecting cancer at an early stage, before it has advanced and spread, greatly improves the chances of successful outcomes and more manageable treatment options. Timely detection allows for prompt intervention, potentially reducing the severity of the disease and improving the overall quality of life for individuals diagnosed with cancer. Here's why early detection and diagnosis are so important:

1. Improved Treatment Options: Cancers that are detected early are often smaller and localized, making them more amenable to a wider range of treatment options. These options may include less invasive surgeries, targeted therapies, and a higher likelihood of successful treatment outcomes.

2. Better Prognosis: When cancer is diagnosed at an early stage, the prognosis is generally more favorable. The likelihood of complete remission, long-term survival, and a better quality of life is significantly enhanced.

3. Reduced Treatment Intensity: Early-stage cancers may require less aggressive and less intensive treatments, leading to fewer side effects and a quicker recovery period. This can help minimize the physical and emotional toll on patients and their families.

4. Minimized Spread: Cancer that is detected and treated early is less likely to have spread to nearby lymph nodes or distant parts of the body. This reduces the risk of metastasis, which can complicate treatment and decrease survival rates.

5. Preservation of Organ Function: Early detection may allow for the preservation of important organ function. For instance, detecting breast cancer at an early stage may enable breast-conserving surgery instead of a full mastectomy.

6. Screening Programs: Regular screening tests for specific cancers, such as mammograms for breast cancer and colonoscopies for colorectal cancer, are designed to detect abnormalities before symptoms develop. Participation in these screening programs can lead to the early detection of cancer and better outcomes.

7. Increased Treatment Success: Some cancers, such as certain types of leukemia and lymphoma, have a higher likelihood of successful treatment when diagnosed early. Early intervention can lead to effective control and management of these diseases.

8. Patient Empowerment: Early detection empowers individuals to take an active role in their health. Being aware of potential symptoms and seeking medical attention promptly can lead to timely diagnosis and better outcomes.

9. Psychosocial Well-being: Early detection can reduce the emotional burden and anxiety associated with a cancer diagnosis. Individuals may feel a greater sense of control and be better prepared for the treatment journey.

10. Reduced Healthcare Costs: Treating cancer at an early stage may lead to lower healthcare costs. Early intervention can prevent the need for more extensive and expensive treatments that may be required at later stages of the disease.

Promoting awareness of the importance of early detection, participating in recommended screening programs, and promptly seeking medical attention for concerning symptoms are crucial steps individuals can take to contribute to their own health and well-being. Healthcare providers, public health organizations, and communities play a pivotal role in advocating for early detection and ensuring that individuals have access to appropriate screening and diagnostic services. Early detection not only saves lives but also empowers individuals to proactively manage their health and take control of their cancer journey.

3.1 Importance of Regular Screenings and Checkups

Regular screenings and checkups are fundamental components of proactive healthcare that play a crucial role in maintaining overall well-being and preventing or detecting diseases, including cancer, at early and more treatable stages. These routine medical evaluations offer numerous benefits for individuals of all ages, helping them stay healthy, identify potential health concerns, and make informed decisions about their health. Here's why regular screenings and checkups are of utmost importance:

1. Early Detection of Diseases: Regular screenings are designed to detect health issues before symptoms appear. Detecting diseases, including cancer, in their early stages often leads to more successful treatment outcomes and can significantly improve prognosis and quality of life.

2. Cancer Prevention: Many cancers can be detected through screenings before symptoms develop. Mammograms, colonoscopies, Pap smears, and prostate-specific antigen (PSA) tests are examples of screenings that can identify cancer at an early, more treatable stage, reducing the risk of advanced disease.

3. Risk Assessment: Regular checkups allow healthcare providers to assess an individual's risk factors for various health conditions, including genetic predispositions and lifestyle factors. This assessment enables personalized recommendations for prevention and early intervention.

4. Chronic Disease Management: Regular checkups are essential for managing chronic conditions like diabetes, hypertension, and heart disease. Monitoring these conditions helps prevent complications and allows for adjustments to treatment plans as needed.

5. Medication Management: Checkups provide an opportunity to review and adjust medications, ensuring that prescribed treatments are effective and appropriate for an individual's current health status.

6. Preventive Services: Routine checkups offer a chance to receive preventive services such as vaccinations, screenings, and counseling on healthy behaviors. These services are essential for disease prevention and overall health promotion.

7. Lifestyle Guidance: Healthcare providers can offer guidance on maintaining a healthy lifestyle, including recommendations for diet, exercise, stress management, and tobacco and alcohol use. These recommendations can have a positive impact on health and longevity.

8. Detection of Silent Conditions: Some health conditions, such as high blood pressure or high cholesterol, may not cause noticeable symptoms. Regular checkups help detect these "silent"conditions, enabling early management to prevent complications.

9. Establishing a Health Baseline: Regular screenings and checkups create a baseline for an individual's health status over time. This baseline allows healthcare providers to identify changes and trends that may indicate potential health concerns.

10. Peace of Mind: Consistent screenings and checkups offer peace of mind, as individuals can be confident in their health status and address any potential issues promptly. This proactive approach reduces anxiety and empowers individuals to take control of their well-being.

11. Healthcare Continuity: Establishing a relationship with a primary care provider through regular checkups ensures continuity of care. This provider can coordinate various aspects of an individual's health and refer to specialists if needed.

3.2 Diagnostic Tools and Techniques

Advancements in medical science have led to a wide array of sophisticated diagnostic tools and techniques that play a pivotal role in identifying, diagnosing, and monitoring various medical conditions, including cancer. These tools have revolutionized healthcare by enabling earlier and more accurate diagnoses, guiding treatment decisions, and improving patient outcomes. Here is an overview of some of the key diagnostic tools and techniques used in modern medicine:

1. Imaging Modalities

A. X-rays: X-ray imaging uses ionizing radiation to create detailed images of bones and certain tissues, helping diagnose fractures, infections, and lung conditions.

B. Computed Tomography (CT) Scan: CT scans produce cross-sectional images of the body, providing detailed views of internal structures. They are used to diagnose a range of conditions, including cancer, cardiovascular issues, and trauma.

C. Magnetic Resonance Imaging (MRI): MRI uses powerful magnets and radio waves to create detailed images of soft tissues and organs. It is particularly useful for diagnosing neurological, musculoskeletal, and abdominal conditions.

 D. Ultrasound: Ultrasound uses high-frequency sound waves to create real-time images of organs and tissues. It is commonly used for imaging the abdomen, pelvis, and during pregnancy.
E. Positron Emission Tomography (PET) Scan: PET scans involve injecting a small amount of radioactive

material to visualize metabolic activity within the body. They are valuable for cancer staging and monitoring treatment response.

2. Laboratory Tests

A. Blood Tests: Blood tests measure various components, including blood cell counts, electrolytes, and specific biomarkers. They help diagnose conditions like anemia, infections, and hormonal imbalances.

B. Biopsy: A biopsy involves collecting tissue samples for examination under a microscope. It is a crucial diagnostic tool for cancer and other conditions.

3. Endoscopy

A. Colonoscopy: Colonoscopy uses a flexible tube with a camera to examine the colon and rectum, aiding in the detection of polyps, tumors, and inflammation.

B. Bronchoscopy: Bronchoscopy allows visualization of the airways and lungs, aiding in diagnosing lung conditions and obtaining tissue samples.

4. Genetic Testing

A. Molecular Diagnostics: Genetic tests analyze DNA, RNA, and proteins to identify genetic mutations, assess disease risk, and guide treatment decisions. They are increasingly used in personalized medicine approaches.

5. Nuclear Medicine

A. Single Photon Emission Computed Tomography (SPECT): SPECT scans provide three-dimensional images of blood flow, organ function, and other physiological processes.

B. Gamma Camera: Gamma camera scans track the distribution of a radioactive tracer within the body to diagnose conditions like thyroid disorders and bone metastases.

6. Biomedical Imaging

A. Fluorescence Imaging: Fluorescence-based techniques use fluorescent dyes to visualize specific molecules, cells, or tissues. They have applications in cancer surgery and research.

7. Telemedicine and Digital Health

A . Telehealth: Telehealth utilizes technology to facilitate remote consultations, diagnostics, and monitoring of patients, especially useful in providing healthcare access to underserved or remote areas. These diagnostic tools and techniques enable healthcare professionals to make informed decisions about patient care, personalize treatment plans, and monitor disease progression. Their continued development and integration into healthcare practice contribute to earlier interventions, improved patient outcomes, and the advancement of medical knowledge.

3.3 Recognizing Warning Signs and Symptoms

Being able to recognize warning signs and symptoms of various health conditions, including cancer, is a crucial skill that empowers individuals to seek timely medical attention and intervention. Early detection plays a pivotal role in improving treatment outcomes and enhancing the overall quality of life. Understanding common warning signs and symptoms can lead to prompt diagnosis, effective management, and potentially life-saving interventions. Here's an overview of why recognizing warning signs and symptoms is essential:

1. Early Detection: Many health conditions, including cancer, are more treatable when detected at an early stage. Being aware of warning signs allows individuals to seek medical evaluation promptly, increasing the chances of early intervention and successful treatment.

2. Preventive Action: Recognizing symptoms early may enable individuals to make lifestyle modifications or seek medical guidance to prevent the progression of a condition. Taking proactive steps can contribute to better health outcomes and reduce the risk of complications.

3. Quality of Life: Timely recognition and management of symptoms can improve an individual's overall quality of life. Addressing discomfort, pain, or other symptoms promptly helps alleviate suffering and improve well-being.

4. Diagnostic Accuracy: Providing healthcare professionals with accurate information about symptoms can aid in the diagnostic process. Clear communication enables doctors to make informed decisions regarding tests, screenings, and further evaluation.

5. Timely Treatment: Early recognition of symptoms allows for prompt initiation of appropriate treatment. This is particularly important for conditions that can worsen rapidly if left untreated.

6. Avoiding Progression: Ignoring warning signs can lead to the progression of a condition, potentially making it more challenging to treat. Addressing symptoms early can help prevent complications and limit the impact of the disease.

7. Patient Empowerment: Recognizing symptoms empowers individuals to take an active role in their health. It encourages them to seek medical advice, advocate for themselves, and make informed decisions about their care.

8. Reduced Healthcare Costs: Detecting health issues at an early stage may result in less complex and costly interventions. Preventing the need for extensive treatments or hospitalizations can lead to reduced healthcare expenses.

9. Educational Awareness: Being knowledgeable about warning signs and symptoms allows individuals to educate their friends and family. This contributes to a collective understanding of health and encourages others to seek medical attention when needed.

10. Engagement in Screening Programs: Recognizing symptoms may prompt individuals to participate in recommended screening programs. Regular screenings can detect conditions before symptoms arise, leading to even earlier intervention.

Common warning signs and symptoms that should prompt further medical evaluation include unexplained weight loss, persistent pain, changes in bowel or bladder habits, chronic fatigue, difficulty swallowing, skin changes, persistent coughing or hoarseness, and unusual bleeding. It's essential to remember that some conditions may be asymptomatic or have subtle symptoms, highlighting the importance of regular checkups and screenings.

By being attentive to their bodies and seeking medical attention when warning signs arise, individuals can take a proactive approach to their health. This vigilance can lead to early diagnosis, effective treatment, and improved overall well-being.

Chapter 4

Conventional Cancer Treatments

Conventional cancer treatments are widely used medical approaches that have been developed and refined over decades to effectively target and combat cancerous cells. These treatments are rooted in evidence-based medicine and have demonstrated success in treating various types of cancer. While the landscape of cancer treatment is evolving with the emergence of new therapies, conventional treatments remain integral to the fight against cancer. Here's an overview of some of the key conventional cancer treatments:

1. Surgery: Surgery involves the removal of cancerous tumors or tissues from the body. It is often used to remove localized tumors and can be curative if the cancer has not spread.

2. Chemotherapy: Chemotherapy involves the use of drugs to target and destroy cancer cells. It can be administered orally or through intravenous infusion and is often used to treat systemic or metastatic cancers.

3. Radiation Therapy: Radiation therapy uses high-energy rays to target and destroy cancer cells. It can be delivered externally (external beam radiation) or internally (brachytherapy) and is effective in shrinking tumors and preventing their growth.

4. Hormone Therapy: Hormone therapy is used to block or interfere with hormones that fuel certain types of cancer. It is commonly used to treat hormone-sensitive cancers like breast and prostate cancer.

5. Immunotherapy: Immunotherapy stimulates the body's immune system to recognize and attack cancer cells. It includes various approaches such as checkpoint inhibitors, cancer vaccines, and adoptive T-cell therapy.

6. Targeted Therapy: Targeted therapy involves drugs that specifically target molecular or genetic alterations in cancer cells, disrupting their growth and survival. These therapies have fewer side effects compared to traditional chemotherapy.

7.Stem Cell Transplantation: Stem cell transplantation involves replacing damaged bone marrow with healthy stem cells to restore normal blood cell production. It is used to treat certain blood-related cancers and disorders.

8. Precision Medicine: Precision medicine tailors treatment plans based on an individual's genetic makeup and the specific characteristics of their cancer. This approach maximizes treatment effectiveness while minimizing side effects.

9.Combination Therapies: Many cancer treatments are administered in combination to achieve better outcomes. For instance, chemotherapy may be combined with radiation therapy or targeted therapy.

10. Palliative Care: While not curative, palliative care focuses on managing symptoms, improving quality of life, and providing support for patients undergoing cancer treatment.

Conventional cancer treatments are determined based on factors such as the type and stage of cancer, the patient's overall health, and their treatment goals. These treatments have led to significant advancements in cancer care, increasing survival rates and improving the lives of countless patients. It's important to note that advancements continue to occur, and new therapies are constantly being developed to further enhance cancer treatment options.

4.1 Surgery: Types and Considerations

Surgery is a medical procedure that involves cutting into a patient's body to treat a variety of conditions. There are several types of surgeries, each with its own set of considerations and implications.

1. Elective Surgery: These surgeries are planned in advance and are not considered urgent. They are often performed to improve a patient's quality of life, such as cosmetic surgeries or joint replacements.

2. Emergency Surgery: These surgeries are performed urgently, often to save a patient's life or prevent further complications. Examples include appendectomies or surgeries to repair traumatic injuries.

3. Minimally Invasive Surgery: Also known as laparoscopic or keyhole surgery, this approach uses small incisions and specialized tools to minimize damage to surrounding tissues. It typically results in quicker recovery times and less scarring.

4. Open Surgery: In contrast to minimally invasive surgery, open surgery involves larger incisions, providing direct access to the surgical area. It might be necessary for complex procedures or when the surgeon needs a better view and access.

5. Reconstructive Surgery: This type of surgery aims to restore function or appearance to a body part that has been affected due to injury, disease, or congenital abnormalities. It includes procedures like skin grafts or breast reconstruction.

6. Transplant Surgery: Organ or tissue transplantation involves replacing a damaged or malfunctioning organ with a healthy one from a donor. Common transplants include kidneys, hearts, and livers.

7. Orthopedic Surgery: Focused on the musculoskeletal system, orthopedic surgeries address issues with bones, joints, ligaments, tendons, and muscles. Joint replacements and fracture repairs fall under this category.

Considerations for Surgery

1. Risks and Benefits: Patients must weigh the potential benefits of surgery against the associated risks, such as infection, bleeding, or adverse reactions to anesthesia.

2. Preoperative Preparation: This includes medical assessments, tests, and following pre-surgery instructions like fasting. Proper preparation reduces complications.

3. Choice of Surgeon: Selecting a qualified and experienced surgeon is crucial for a successful outcome. Patients should research their surgeon's credentials and ask about their experience with the specific procedure.

4. Anesthesia: The type of anesthesia used (local, regional, general) depends on the surgery and the patient's medical condition. An anesthesiologist evaluates the patient and administers the anesthesia.

5. Recovery and Aftercare: Understanding post-operative care is essential. This includes wound care, medications, physical therapy, and follow-up appointments.

6. Potential Alternatives: In some cases, non-surgical treatments or alternative procedures may be considered before opting for surgery.

7. Cost and Insurance: Patients should be aware of the financial implications of surgery and confirm coverage with their insurance provider.

8. Mental and Emotional Preparation: Surgery can be stressful. Patients should address any concerns or anxieties and have a support system in place.

It's important for patients to have thorough discussions with their healthcare providers to make informed decisions about the type of surgery that best suits their needs and circumstances.

4.2 Chemotherapy: How it Works and Side Effects

Chemotherapy is a widely used medical treatment for cancer that involves the use of powerful drugs to destroy

or slow down the growth of cancer cells. It is one of the key components in the fight against cancer and is often employed in combination with other treatments like surgery, radiation therapy, or targeted therapies.
How Chemotherapy Works

Chemotherapy drugs work by targeting and disrupting the rapid growth and division of cancer cells. They interfere with the cell's ability to divide and multiply, ultimately leading to cell death. Chemotherapy can be administered in different ways:

1. Intravenous (IV): The drugs are injected directly into a vein, allowing them to quickly circulate through the bloodstream to reach cancer cells throughout the body.

2. Oral: Some chemotherapy drugs are available in pill or capsule form and can be taken by mouth.

3. Topical: Certain types of chemotherapy can be applied directly to the skin as creams or ointments for treating skin cancers.

4. Injection: Chemotherapy drugs can be injected into specific body parts, such as the spinal fluid (intrathecal) or muscle tissue (intramuscular).

Side Effects of Chemotherapy
While chemotherapy is effective in targeting cancer cells, it also affects normal, healthy cells that divide rapidly, leading to a range of side effects. The severity and type of side effects vary depending on the specific drugs used, the dosage, the patient's overall health, and the duration of treatment. Common side effects include:

1. Fatigue: Chemotherapy can cause extreme tiredness and lack of energy.

2. Nausea and Vomiting: Many chemotherapy drugs can affect the stomach lining, leading to feelings of nausea and vomiting.

3. Hair Loss: Rapidly dividing hair follicle cells are affected, resulting in hair loss from the scalp and other body parts.

4. Suppressed Immune System: Chemotherapy can weaken the immune system, making patients more susceptible to infections.

5. Anemia: Reduced red blood cell production may lead to anemia, causing fatigue and weakness.

6. Mouth Sores: Chemotherapy can damage the cells lining the mouth and throat, resulting in painful sores.

7. Changes in Appetite and Taste: Some patients experience changes in taste perception and appetite.

8. Skin and Nail Changes: Skin may become dry, itchy, or more sensitive to sunlight. Nails might become brittle or discolored.

9. Nerve Damage: Some chemotherapy drugs can cause peripheral neuropathy, resulting in numbness, tingling, or pain in the extremities.

10. Fertility Issues: Chemotherapy can affect fertility in both men and women.

It's important to note that not all patients will experience the same side effects, and advancements in supportive care have helped in managing and minimizing these effects. Medical professionals closely monitor patients during treatment and can adjust the treatment plan if side effects become too severe. The goal is to strike a balance between effectively targeting cancer cells and maintaining the patient's overall well-being.

4.3 Radiation Therapy: Applications and Innovations

Radiation therapy, also known as radiotherapy, is a crucial medical treatment that employs high doses of targeted radiation to destroy or damage cancer cells. This therapy plays a significant role in cancer treatment and has witnessed several innovative advancements over the years.

Applications of Radiation Therapy

1. Curative Treatment: Radiation therapy can be the primary treatment for certain cancers, aiming to completely eliminate cancer cells and achieve a cure.

2. Adjuvant Treatment: After surgery to remove a tumor, radiation therapy can be used to kill any remaining cancer cells and reduce the risk of recurrence.

3. Palliative Care: Radiation therapy can alleviate symptoms and improve the quality of life for patients with advanced or metastatic cancers by shrinking tumors and reducing pain.

4. Neoadjuvant Treatment: Radiation therapy may be used before surgery to shrink tumors, making them easier to remove.

5. Combination Therapy: It is often used in conjunction with other treatments such as surgery, chemotherapy, and targeted therapy to enhance overall treatment effectiveness.

Innovations in Radiation Therapy

1. Intensity-Modulated Radiation Therapy (IMRT): IMRT delivers precise radiation doses to tumor regions while minimizing exposure to nearby healthy tissues. It uses advanced software to adjust the intensity of the radiation beams.

2. Image-Guided Radiation Therapy (IGRT): IGRT uses real-time imaging techniques, such as X-rays or CT scans, to accurately locate the tumor before each treatment session. This ensures that radiation is precisely directed to the tumor.

3. Stereotactic Radiosurgery (SRS) and Stereotactic Body Radiotherapy (SBRT): These techniques deliver high doses of radiation with extreme precision to small tumors or specific areas, often completed in a few sessions.

4. Proton Therapy: Proton therapy uses protons (charged particles) instead of X-rays to deliver radiation. It can be particularly useful for tumors located near sensitive organs, as it reduces radiation exposure to healthy tissues.

5. Brachytherapy: This involves placing a radiation source directly into or near the tumor. It is used for various cancers, including prostate, cervical, and breast cancer.

6. Particle Therapy: Beyond protons, other particles like heavy ions are being explored for their potential in targeting certain types of cancer cells more effectively.

7. Radiomics and Radiogenomics: These are data-driven approaches that analyze medical images to extract quantitative data about tumors. This information can help personalize treatment plans and predict treatment outcomes.

8. Artificial Intelligence (AI): AI is being employed to assist in treatment planning, tumor tracking, and predicting patient responses to radiation therapy.

9. FLASH Therapy: This experimental technique delivers ultra-high doses of radiation in a fraction of a second, potentially minimizing damage to healthy tissues.

Radiation therapy continues to evolve, becoming more precise, effective, and personalized. These innovations aim to enhance treatment outcomes, reduce side effects, and improve the overall patient experience in the fight against cancer.

Chapter 5

Complementary and Alternative Therapies

Complementary and Alternative Therapies (CAM) encompass a diverse range of healthcare practices and treatments that lie outside the conventional realm of Western medicine. These approaches often focus on holistic well-being, addressing the physical, mental, emotional, and spiritual aspects of health.
CAM therapies can be categorized into various types:

1. Mind-Body Interventions: These therapies emphasize the connection between the mind and body, aiming to promote relaxation, reduce stress, and enhance overall wellness. Examples include meditation, yoga, tai chi, and guided imagery.

2. Herbal and Dietary Supplements: Natural products, such as herbs, vitamins, and minerals, are used to support health and treat specific conditions. However, caution is advised, as some supplements may interact with medications or have unpredictable effects.

3. Manipulative and Body-Based Practices: These involve physical manipulation of the body, often focusing on musculoskeletal issues. Chiropractic care, osteopathy, and massage therapy fall under this category.

4. Energy Therapies: Based on the concept of energy flow within the body, therapies like acupuncture, acupressure, and Reiki aim to balance this energy and promote healing.

5. Traditional and Cultural Practices: Many cultures have their own traditional healing methods, such as Ayurveda, traditional Chinese medicine (TCM), and Indigenous healing practices. These therapies often have a holistic approach, considering the individual's connection to nature and their environment.

6. Mind-Body Practices: Techniques like meditation, mindfulness, and biofeedback help individuals become more attuned to their thoughts, emotions, and bodily sensations, fostering self-awareness and stress reduction.

It's important to note that while some CAM therapies have shown promise in promoting well-being and complementing conventional treatments, others lack scientific evidence and may even pose risks. It's advisable to consult with healthcare professionals before incorporating CAM therapies, especially when dealing with serious medical conditions.

The integration of CAM and conventional medicine, often referred to as "integrative medicine,"has gained popularity in recent years. This approach seeks to combine the strengths of both paradigms, providing patients with a comprehensive and individualized healthcare experience.

Before pursuing any CAM therapy, individuals should:
- Research thoroughly and verify the credentials of practitioners.
- Discuss their intentions with a qualified healthcare provider.
- Be cautious of unsubstantiated claims or promises of a "cure."

- Inform their healthcare team about all therapies and supplements being used.

5.1 Herbal Medicine and Natural Supplements

Herbal Medicine and Natural Supplements have been used for centuries as a means to promote health, treat ailments, and enhance well-being. These remedies are derived from plants, minerals, and other natural sources, and they continue to play a significant role in healthcare practices around the world.

Herbal Medicine

1. History and Tradition: Herbal medicine has deep roots in various cultures, including traditional Chinese medicine, Ayurveda, Native American practices, and European herbalism. Knowledge of plant properties and their effects on the body has been passed down through generations.

2. Plant-Based Remedies: Herbal remedies often involve the use of specific parts of plants, such as leaves, roots, flowers, or seeds. These parts contain bioactive compounds that can have therapeutic effects on the body.

3. Holistic Approach: Herbal medicine considers the whole person and aims to address the underlying causes of illness rather than just alleviating symptoms. It emphasizes the balance and harmony of the body's systems.

4. Safety and Caution: While many herbs are considered safe, some can interact with medications or cause adverse reactions. It's crucial to consult with a knowledgeable healthcare professional before using herbal remedies, especially if you have pre-existing health conditions.

5. Common Herbal Remedies: Examples of widely used herbs include Echinacea for immune support, St. John's Wort for mood management, and ginger for digestion. Chamomile and valerian are often used for relaxation and sleep.

Natural Supplements

1. Vitamins and Minerals: Natural supplements encompass a wide range of products, including vitamins (e.g., vitamin C, vitamin D) and minerals (e.g., calcium, magnesium). These micronutrients are essential for various bodily functions.

2. Health and Wellness Support: Natural supplements are commonly used to fill nutritional gaps in the diet and support overall health. For example, omega-3 fatty acids are known for their cardiovascular benefits.

3. Joint and Bone Health: Supplements like glucosamine and chondroitin are often taken to support joint health, while calcium and vitamin D are crucial for maintaining strong bones.

4. Sports Performance: Athletes may use natural supplements like protein powders, creatine, and branched-chain amino acids (BCAAs) to enhance performance, aid recovery, and build muscle.

5. Cautions and Considerations: While natural supplements can provide benefits, they should be used judiciously. Overuse or reliance on supplements as a substitute for a balanced diet can have negative consequences.

Key Considerations

1. Quality and Regulation: It's important to choose reputable brands that adhere to quality standards and have their products tested by third-party organizations.

2. Dosage and Guidance: Following recommended dosages and guidelines is crucial to ensure safety and effectiveness.

3. Personalization: Not all supplements are suitable for everyone. Factors such as age, gender, health status, and lifestyle should be taken into account.

5.2 Acupuncture and Traditional Chinese Medicine (TCM)

Acupuncture and Traditional Chinese Medicine (TCM) are ancient healing practices that have been integral parts of Chinese culture for thousands of years. Rooted in a holistic understanding of the body and its energy systems, these practices continue to gain recognition and popularity worldwide for their potential to promote health and alleviate various ailments.

Acupuncture

1. Principle of Qi: Acupuncture is based on the concept of "Qi"(pronounced "chee"), which refers to the vital energy that flows through pathways known as meridians in the body. When Qi is balanced and flowing smoothly, health is maintained; disruptions in this flow can lead to illness.

2. Fine Needles: Acupuncture involves the insertion of fine, sterile needles into specific points along the body's meridians. These points are believed to correspond to different organs and systems, and stimulating them is thought to restore the flow of Qi.

3. Pain Management: Acupuncture is commonly used to manage pain, including chronic pain conditions such as back pain, migraines, and arthritis. It's believed that acupuncture can stimulate the release of endorphins and other natural pain-relieving substances.

4. Holistic Approach: Acupuncture practitioners consider the individual as a whole, addressing not only physical symptoms but also emotional and mental well-being. This holistic perspective contributes to its effectiveness in treating a wide range of conditions.

5. Research and Integration: While the mechanisms of acupuncture are still being studied, research has shown promising results in various areas, such as pain relief, stress reduction, and even fertility support. Acupuncture is increasingly being integrated into conventional medical settings.

Traditional Chinese Medicine (TCM)

1. Holistic Philosophy: TCM is a comprehensive system of medicine that encompasses various modalities, including acupuncture, herbal medicine, dietary therapy, and exercise (e.g., Tai Chi and Qigong). It is rooted in the belief that health results from the balance of Yin and Yang energies and the harmonious flow of Qi.

2. Diagnostic Techniques: TCM diagnosis involves assessing a person's constitution, observing physical symptoms, and analyzing factors such as pulse and tongue appearance. Patterns of disharmony are identified, and treatments are tailored accordingly.

3. Herbal Medicine: Herbal remedies play a significant role in TCM. Herbs are combined in formulas to address specific patterns of imbalance. These formulas can be taken internally as teas, powders, or pills.

4. Preventive Care: TCM places great emphasis on preventive care and maintaining balance within the body. Adjusting one's lifestyle, diet, and daily habits according to TCM principles can help prevent illness.

5. Chronic Conditions: TCM is often sought for chronic conditions that may not respond well to conventional treatments alone, such as digestive disorders, insomnia, and anxiety.

6. Global Influence: TCM's influence has extended beyond China, with practitioners and clinics offering TCM therapies worldwide. However, it's important to seek treatment from qualified and trained practitioners.

5.3 Mind-Body Techniques: Meditation and Yoga

Mind-body techniques encompass a range of practices that emphasize the interconnectedness of the mind and body, promoting holistic well-being and fostering a sense of inner calm and balance. Two prominent practices within this realm are meditation and yoga.

Meditation

1. Inner Awareness: Meditation is a practice that involves focusing the mind and eliminating distractions to achieve a heightened state of awareness and mental clarity. It encourages a non-judgmental observation of thoughts, emotions, and sensations.

2. Stress Reduction: One of the primary benefits of meditation is its ability to reduce stress and anxiety. Regular practice can help individuals manage their reactions to stressors and cultivate a greater sense of calm.

3. Mindfulness: Mindfulness meditation, a popular form of meditation, involves being fully present in the moment and observing one's thoughts without attachment. It has been integrated into various therapeutic settings and has shown positive effects on mental well-being.

4. Concentration and Focus: Meditation techniques often involve focusing attention on a specific object, sound, or breath. This can enhance concentration, attention span, and cognitive function.

5. Health Benefits: Research suggests that meditation can have physiological benefits, such as reducing blood pressure, improving sleep, and boosting the immune system.

Yoga

1. Physical and Mental Union: Yoga is a holistic practice that combines physical postures (asanas), breathing techniques (pranayama), and meditation to cultivate a balanced and harmonious connection between the body, mind, and spirit.

2. Flexibility and Strength: The physical postures in yoga promote flexibility, balance, and strength. Regular practice can enhance body awareness and posture.

3. Stress Relief: Yoga's focus on mindful movement and breathwork helps reduce stress by activating the body's relaxation response and calming the nervous system.

4. Mindful Movement: Many forms of yoga emphasize the mindful execution of movements, fostering a deep connection between the breath and body. This encourages a state of presence and self-awareness.

5. Variety of Styles: There are various styles of yoga, from gentle and restorative to more vigorous and dynamic. Each style offers unique benefits and can be adapted to different fitness levels and preferences.

6. Holistic Health: Yoga's philosophy extends beyond the physical practice, encouraging ethical and moral principles that contribute to a balanced and purposeful life.

7. Research and Integration: The therapeutic benefits of yoga have gained recognition in the medical field, leading to its integration into complementary healthcare settings and rehabilitation programs.

Chapter 6

Integrative Cancer Care

Integrative Cancer Care is an approach that combines conventional medical treatments with complementary and alternative therapies to provide a comprehensive and holistic approach to cancer treatment and management. It recognizes that cancer care extends beyond medical interventions, aiming to address the physical, emotional, and spiritual needs of individuals facing a cancer diagnosis.

Key Components of Integrative Cancer Care

1. Collaborative Approach: Integrative cancer care involves a multidisciplinary team of healthcare professionals, including medical doctors, oncologists, naturopathic doctors, nutritionists, therapists, and more. These experts collaborate to develop a personalized treatment plan that integrates both conventional and complementary therapies.

2. Complementary Therapies: Complementary therapies such as acupuncture, massage therapy, yoga, meditation, and nutritional counseling are used alongside conventional treatments to support overall well-being, reduce treatment side effects, and enhance quality of life.

3. Nutritional Support: Nutrition plays a crucial role in cancer care. Integrative approaches emphasize a balanced and nourishing diet tailored to support the individual's specific needs and treatment regimen.

4. Mind-Body Techniques: Mind-body practices like meditation, mindfulness, and relaxation techniques can help manage stress, anxiety, and depression that often accompany a cancer diagnosis.

5. Herbal and Natural Supplements: Some integrative cancer care plans may incorporate herbal remedies and natural supplements to support the body's immune system, reduce inflammation, and manage treatment side effects.

6. Exercise and Physical Activity: Regular physical activity is encouraged as part of integrative cancer care. Exercise can help maintain strength, improve mood, and enhance overall well-being during and after treatment.

7. Emotional and Psychological Support: Integrative cancer care addresses the emotional and psychological aspects of cancer by providing counseling, support groups, and therapies to help individuals cope with the challenges of diagnosis, treatment, and survivorship.

8. Spiritual Care: Recognizing the importance of spirituality for some individuals, integrative cancer care may offer spiritual guidance and practices that align with the individual's beliefs.

Benefits of Integrative Cancer Care

1. Enhanced Quality of Life: Integrative approaches can improve physical, emotional, and mental well-being, leading to a better quality of life for cancer patients and survivors.

2. Reduced Treatment Side Effects: Complementary therapies can help manage treatment-related side effects such as pain, nausea, fatigue, and sleep disturbances.

3. Empowerment: Integrative cancer care empowers patients by involving them in the decision-making process and providing them with a range of tools to actively participate in their treatment and recovery.

4. Holistic Healing: By addressing various aspects of a person's health, integrative cancer care promotes holistic healing and encourages a sense of balance and harmony.

5. Personalized Approach: Integrative cancer care recognizes that each individual's experience with cancer is unique. Treatment plans are tailored to the person's specific needs, preferences, and goals.

6.1 Combining Conventional and Alternative Approaches to Healthcare

In recent years, there has been a growing recognition of the potential benefits of combining conventional medical treatments with alternative and complementary therapies. This integrative approach aims to provide a comprehensive and personalized approach to healthcare, addressing not only physical symptoms but also emotional, mental, and spiritual well-being. By blending the strengths of both paradigms, individuals can access a broader range of tools to enhance their health and healing.

Key Principles of Integrating Conventional and Alternative Approaches

1. Holistic Well-being: Integrative care recognizes that health is a complex interplay of various factors, including physical, emotional, social, and environmental aspects. By addressing the whole person, this approach aims to promote holistic well-being.

2. Collaboration: Effective integration involves close collaboration between conventional healthcare providers and qualified practitioners of alternative therapies. This ensures that treatments are coordinated, safe, and complementary.

3. Personalization: Each person's health journey is unique. Integrative care tailors treatments and therapies to the individual's specific needs, preferences, and goals.

4. Evidence-Based Practice: Integrative care combines therapies that have a solid scientific foundation with those that have shown promise in improving well-being. This helps ensure that the approach is both safe and effective.

5. Informed Decision-Making: Integrative care encourages individuals to be active participants in their healthcare decisions. It provides them with information about the available options, empowering them to make informed choices.

Examples of Combining Conventional and Alternative Approaches

1. Cancer Treatment: Integrative cancer care may involve combining chemotherapy or radiation with complementary therapies such as acupuncture, massage, meditation, and nutritional counseling to manage treatment side effects and improve overall well-being.

2. Chronic Pain Management: Conventional pain medications could be supplemented with therapies like chiropractic care, physical therapy, and mindfulness meditation to manage pain and improve mobility.

3. Mental Health: Conventional therapies like medication and psychotherapy could be complemented with yoga, art therapy, and herbal supplements to support emotional and mental well-being.

4. Cardiovascular Health: For heart health, a combination of medication, dietary changes, and exercise could be complemented with stress-reduction techniques like meditation and biofeedback.

5. Chronic Illness: For conditions like diabetes, conventional medical management could be combined with dietary adjustments, herbal supplements, and stress-reduction techniques to optimize health outcomes.

Benefits of Combining Approaches

1. Enhanced Results: Integrating conventional and alternative approaches can lead to improved treatment outcomes and better symptom management.

2. Reduced Side Effects: Complementary therapies can help mitigate side effects of conventional treatments, enhancing overall comfort.

3. Empowerment: Integrative care empowers individuals to take an active role in their health, leading to a sense of ownership and engagement in the healing process.

4. Personal Satisfaction: Many individuals find satisfaction in being able to explore a range of treatment options and actively contribute to their well-being.

Considerations

A. Consult with qualified healthcare professionals before integrating alternative therapies, especially if you have pre-existing health conditions or are on medications.

B. Open communication between conventional healthcare providers and alternative practitioners is crucial to ensure safety and effectiveness.

C. Make informed choices based on credible information and evidence.

6.2 Integrating Emotional and Psychological Support into Healthcare

Recognizing the intrinsic link between emotional well-being and physical health, the integration of emotional and psychological support into healthcare has become increasingly important. This holistic approach acknowledges that mental and emotional factors significantly impact overall health outcomes, and it seeks to provide comprehensive care that addresses both the physical and emotional needs of individuals.

Key Aspects of Integrating Emotional and Psychological Support

1. Holistic Perspective: Integrative healthcare understands that emotional well-being is integral to overall health. It acknowledges that emotional distress can exacerbate physical conditions and vice versa.

2. Collaborative Care: Effective integration involves collaboration between healthcare professionals from various disciplines, such as medical doctors, psychologists, counselors, and social workers. This team approach ensures that all aspects of an individual's well-being are considered.

3. Early Intervention: Identifying and addressing emotional and psychological needs early can prevent the development of more serious mental health issues and contribute to better overall outcomes.

4. Patient-Centered Care: Integrative care places the individual at the center, valuing their preferences, needs, and goals. It encourages open communication and shared decision-making.

Examples of Integrating Emotional and Psychological Support

1. Chronic Illness Management: Individuals with chronic conditions like diabetes or heart disease may receive emotional support to cope with the challenges of managing their conditions, reduce stress, and improve adherence to treatment plans.

2. Cancer Care: Emotional and psychological support is often integrated into cancer treatment to help patients manage anxiety, depression, and the emotional impact of diagnosis and treatment.

3. Pain Management: Chronic pain management may involve not only physical interventions but also counseling, cognitive-behavioral therapy, and relaxation techniques to address the emotional aspects of pain.

4. Maternal Health: Pregnancy and postpartum care may include emotional support to address mood disorders, stress, and the emotional adjustments that come with becoming a parent.

Benefits of Integrating Emotional and Psychological Support

1. Improved Well-being: Integrative care contributes to overall well-being by addressing emotional needs, reducing stress, and enhancing mental resilience.

2. Enhanced Treatment Outcomes: Emotional well-being positively influences physical health outcomes, leading to better treatment responses and improved recovery.

3. Preventive Care: Addressing emotional and psychological needs early can prevent the development of mental health disorders and contribute to long-term emotional resilience.

4. Empowerment: Providing emotional support empowers individuals to actively engage in their health journey, leading to better self-management and treatment adherence.

Considerations

A. A patient's emotional and psychological needs should be assessed regularly and incorporated into their care plan.

B. Open communication between healthcare providers and patients is essential to understand emotional challenges and tailor support accordingly.

C. Collaboration between different healthcare professionals ensures a comprehensive and coordinated approach.

6.3 Creating a personalized treatment plan

Creating a personalized treatment plan is a crucial step in providing effective care and support for individuals facing various health challenges. This tailored approach takes into consideration a person's unique medical history, current condition, preferences, and goals.
The process begins with a comprehensive assessment conducted by healthcare professionals. They gather detailed information about the individual's medical history, lifestyle, symptoms, and any relevant diagnostic tests. This data forms the foundation for crafting a treatment plan that addresses the specific needs of the patient.

Healthcare providers collaborate to design a personalized roadmap for treatment. This may involve a combination of therapies, medications, lifestyle adjustments, and interventions. The aim is to target the root causes of the health issue, manage symptoms, and enhance overall well-being.

Regular monitoring and adjustments are integral to the success of the treatment plan. Healthcare providers track the patient's progress, making modifications as needed based on how the individual responds to the interventions. Open communication between the patient and the healthcare team is essential to ensure the plan remains effective and aligned with the patient's goals.

Moreover, a personalized treatment plan considers the patient's preferences and values. It respects their choices and encourages active participation in their healthcare journey. This collaborative approach fosters a sense of empowerment and motivation, which are vital for achieving positive outcomes.

Chapter 7

Promising Advances in Cancer Research

Cancer research has made significant strides in recent years, with promising advances that offer hope for improved treatments and better outcomes for patients. From innovative therapies to advanced diagnostic tools, the field of cancer research is continually evolving and providing new avenues for tackling this complex and devastating disease.

One of the most promising advances in cancer research is the development of immunotherapy treatments. These therapies harness the body's own immune system to target and destroy cancer cells. Immune checkpoint inhibitors, for example, have shown remarkable success in treating certain types of cancer, such as melanoma and lung cancer. By blocking the proteins that inhibit the immune response, these drugs allow the immune system to recognize and attack cancer cells more effectively.

Another exciting development is the use of precision medicine to tailor treatments to each individual patient. Advances in genetic sequencing have enabled researchers to identify specific mutations and genetic markers that drive cancer growth. This information allows doctors to develop personalized treatment plans that target the specific molecular changes driving the disease. Precision medicine has already led to improved outcomes in some cases, and ongoing research aims to expand its applications to a wider range of cancer types. Early detection is also a crucial area of advancement in cancer research. New screening techniques, such as liquid biopsies, can detect tiny fragments of tumor DNA in the blood, allowing for the detection of cancer at its earliest stages. This is particularly important for cancers that are often diagnosed at advanced stages, such as pancreatic and ovarian cancer. By catching these cancers early, patients have a better chance of successful treatment and improved survival rates.

In addition to treatment and detection, researchers are also making strides in understanding the underlying biology of cancer. This knowledge is leading to the development of targeted therapies that exploit specific vulnerabilities in cancer cells. For example, researchers have identified drugs that target cancer cell metabolism, effectively starving the cells of the nutrients they need to grow and survive.

Furthermore, advancements in cancer research are not limited to traditional treatments. Nanotechnology is a rapidly growing field that holds great promise for cancer therapy. Nanoparticles can be engineered to deliver targeted treatments directly to cancer cells, minimizing damage to healthy tissue and reducing side effects. This approach has the potential to revolutionize cancer treatment by making therapies more effective and less toxic.

7.1 Immunotherapy: Harnessing the Immune System for Cancer Treatment

Immunotherapy has emerged as a groundbreaking approach in cancer treatment, offering new hope for patients by harnessing the power of the immune system to fight off the disease. Unlike traditional treatments such as chemotherapy and radiation, which directly target cancer cells, immunotherapy focuses on boosting the body's natural defense mechanisms to recognize and destroy cancer cells more effectively.

The immune system is a complex network of cells, tissues, and organs that work together to defend the body against harmful invaders, such as bacteria, viruses, and cancer cells. In the case of cancer, the immune system often fails to recognize the abnormal cells as a threat, allowing them to proliferate and spread unchecked. Immunotherapy aims to overcome this evasion by enhancing the immune response and training it to target cancer cells specifically.

One of the most well-known types of immunotherapy is immune checkpoint inhibitors. These drugs block the proteins on the surface of cancer cells that inhibit the immune response. By doing so, they unleash the immune system to recognize and attack cancer cells.

Immune checkpoint inhibitors have shown remarkable success in treating a variety of cancer types, including melanoma, lung cancer, and bladder cancer, leading to long-lasting remissions and improved survival rates. Another form of immunotherapy is adoptive T cell therapy, where immune cells called T cells are extracted from the patient's body and genetically modified to target cancer cells. These modified T cells are then infused back into the patient, where they can recognize and eliminate cancer cells. This approach has shown remarkable success in treating certain blood cancers, such as leukemia and lymphoma.

Cancer vaccines are also a promising avenue of immunotherapy. These vaccines stimulate the immune system to recognize and attack cancer cells by presenting them with fragments of tumor proteins. While cancer vaccines are still in the early stages of development, they hold great potential for preventing cancer recurrence and improving long-term outcomes. Furthermore, researchers are exploring the use of oncolytic viruses in immunotherapy. These viruses are engineered to selectively infect and kill cancer cells while leaving healthy cells unharmed. As the cancer cells are destroyed, they release tumor antigens that stimulate the immune system to mount a response against the remaining cancer cells.

While immunotherapy has shown remarkable success in some cases, it is important to note that not all patients will respond to these treatments. Researchers are working tirelessly to understand why some patients benefit while others do not, and ongoing clinical trials are exploring combination therapies and novel approaches to enhance the effectiveness of immunotherapy.

Immunotherapy represents a paradigm shift in cancer treatment, offering a more targeted and less toxic approach compared to traditional therapies. As researchers continue to unlock the complexities of the immune system and develop new strategies for harnessing its power, the future of cancer treatment looks increasingly promising. While challenges remain, the progress made in immunotherapy gives hope to countless patients and their families, offering a brighter outlook in the fight against cancer.

7.2 Targeted Therapies: Precision Medicine in Cancer Treatment

Advancements in cancer research have led to a revolutionary approach in the field of cancer treatment known as targeted therapies. These therapies, also referred to as precision medicine, aim to tailor treatments to the specific genetic and molecular characteristics of a patient's cancer. By identifying and targeting the unique vulnerabilities of cancer cells, targeted therapies offer a more effective and personalized approach to cancer treatment.

Unlike traditional chemotherapy, which attacks both cancerous and healthy cells, targeted therapies focus exclusively on the genetic and molecular alterations that drive the growth and spread of cancer. These alterations can include mutations, overexpressed proteins, and other specific changes that are unique to each patient's tumor. By targeting these specific features, targeted therapies can inhibit the growth of cancer cells while minimizing damage to healthy tissues.

One of the most well-known examples of targeted therapy is the use of tyrosine kinase inhibitors (TKIs) in treating certain types of cancer, such as lung cancer and leukemia. TKIs block the activity of specific proteins that promote cancer growth, effectively shutting down the signals that drive the disease. These drugs have shown impressive results in terms of tumor shrinkage and improved survival rates for patients with certain genetic mutations.

Another approach to targeted therapy is the use of monoclonal antibodies, which are designed to target and bind to specific proteins on the surface of cancer cells. By binding to these proteins, monoclonal antibodies can block the signals that promote cancer growth or trigger the immune system to attack cancer cells. This approach has been successful in treating cancers such as breast cancer and lymphoma.

In addition to these approaches, researchers are also exploring targeted therapies that focus on the tumor microenvironment the surrounding tissue and cells that support cancer growth. By disrupting the interactions between cancer cells and their microenvironment, these therapies can inhibit tumor growth and spread.

Precision medicine also plays a crucial role in overcoming drug resistance, a common challenge in cancer treatment. As cancer cells evolve and adapt to therapies, they can develop resistance to targeted treatments. By continuously monitoring a patient's tumor and its genetic changes, doctors can adjust treatment plans and switch to alternative targeted therapies to overcome drug resistance and continue effectively targeting the cancer.

While targeted therapies hold great promise, it's important to note that not all patients will benefit from these treatments. The success of targeted therapies depends on the specific genetic and molecular characteristics of each patient's cancer. Researchers are working diligently to identify biomarkers and develop predictive tests that can help determine which patients are most likely to respond to targeted therapies.

7.3 Gene Therapy: Unlocking Potential and Confronting Challenges

Gene therapy, a revolutionary medical approach, holds the promise of treating and even curing a wide range of genetic and acquired diseases by manipulating the genetic code within our cells. This groundbreaking field has captured the imagination of researchers, clinicians, and patients alike, offering hope for conditions that were once considered untreatable. However, along with its potential, gene therapy also presents significant challenges that demand careful consideration and innovation.

The Potential

1. Targeted Treatments: Gene therapy allows for precise targeting of underlying genetic causes of diseases, potentially eliminating the need for lifelong medications or invasive treatments.

2. Genetic Disorders: Disorders caused by a single gene mutation, such as cystic fibrosis, muscular dystrophy, and sickle cell anemia, could be effectively addressed through gene therapy.

3. Cancer Treatment: Gene therapy has the potential to reprogram cancer cells, making them more susceptible to the body's immune response or directly killing them.

4. Neurological Diseases: Genetic defects contributing to neurodegenerative disorders like Parkinson's or Alzheimer's could be corrected using gene therapy, offering renewed hope for patients.

The Challenges

1. Delivery Systems: Efficiently delivering therapeutic genes into target cells remains a major hurdle. Viruses are often used as vectors, but immune responses and potential insertional mutagenesis raise safety concerns.

2. Long-term Effects: Ensuring the stability and safety of introduced genetic modifications over a patient's lifetime is complex, as unintended consequences may arise years after treatment.

3. Immune Response: The body's immune system might react to the therapeutic genes or vectors, potentially reducing the treatment's effectiveness and causing adverse effects.

4. Ethical Considerations: Gene editing of embryos or germline cells raises ethical questions about altering future generations' genetic makeup and unintended consequences.

5. Cost and Accessibility: Developing and administering gene therapies can be expensive, limiting access for many patients and straining healthcare systems.

As researchers continue to refine techniques and understand the intricacies of gene therapy, collaboration between the scientific community, regulators, and industry is essential to navigate these challenges. Rigorous clinical trials, transparent reporting, and ongoing monitoring of patients are critical to ensure the safety and efficacy of gene therapies.

Chapter 8

Empowering Cancer Survivorship: Navigating the Journey with Support

Cancer survivorship marks a momentous achievement in the lives of individuals who have battled the formidable adversary of cancer. Beyond the completion of treatment, survivorship presents its own unique set of challenges and triumphs. The journey from diagnosis to remission is often arduous, encompassing physical, emotional, and psychological dimensions. In this transformative phase, comprehensive support systems play a pivotal role in guiding survivors toward a life of renewed hope and well-being.

The Road to Survivorship

1. Physical Recovery: Cancer treatments can leave survivors with a range of physical challenges, including fatigue, pain, and diminished physical functioning. Post-treatment care focuses on rehabilitation and restoring physical health to help survivors regain their strength and vitality.

2. Emotional Resilience: The emotional toll of cancer can be profound, leading to anxiety, depression, or post-traumatic stress. Survivorship support addresses these psychological aspects, providing counseling, therapy, and coping strategies to enhance emotional well-being.

3. Rebuilding Identity: Many survivors grapple with redefining themselves post-cancer. Support groups and counseling can aid in reestablishing a sense of identity and purpose, allowing survivors to find new meaning and direction in their lives.

The Role of Support Systems

1. Medical Follow-up: Regular medical check-ups and surveillance are crucial during survivorship to monitor for any recurrence or late effects of treatment. Oncology teams play a critical role in overseeing survivors' ongoing health and addressing any concerns.

2. Support Groups: Connecting with fellow survivors fosters a sense of camaraderie and understanding. Sharing experiences, fears, and triumphs in a supportive environment can alleviate feelings of isolation and provide invaluable insights.

3. Lifestyle Guidance: Adopting a healthy lifestyle post-cancer can enhance overall well-being. Nutritional counseling, exercise programs, and stress management techniques empower survivors to make informed choices for their health.

4. Family and Caregiver Involvement: Survivorship affects not only the individual but also their loved ones. Support extends to family members and caregivers, acknowledging their role and providing resources to cope with caregiving-related challenges.

Challenges and Triumphs

1. Fear of Recurrence: The fear of cancer recurrence is a common concern among survivors. Support programs address this fear by providing education, coping mechanisms, and strategies to manage anxiety.

2. Financial and Practical Considerations: The financial burden of cancer can extend beyond treatment. Survivorship support may offer guidance on managing medical bills, insurance, and returning to work or daily routines.

3. Celebrating Milestones: Survivorship milestones, such as anniversaries of remission or completion of treatment, provide opportunities to reflect and celebrate achievements. Support networks can organize events to acknowledge and commemorate these important moments.

Cancer survivorship embodies strength, resilience, and the triumph of the human spirit. The journey is marked by challenges, but with the right support, survivors can embrace life anew. By fostering comprehensive support systems that address physical, emotional, and practical needs, we can empower cancer survivors to navigate the path of survivorship with grace, resilience, and a renewed sense of purpose.

8.1 Life After Cancer: Navigating Coping and Adjustment

Surviving cancer is a monumental achievement, marking the end of a challenging and often grueling journey. However, the transition to life after cancer presents its own set of emotional, physical, and psychological complexities. Coping with the aftermath of treatment and adjusting to a "new normal"can be a transformative process, requiring resilience, support, and self-discovery.

1. Emotional Rollercoaster: The post-cancer period is characterized by a range of emotions, including relief, joy, anxiety, and uncertainty. Survivors may experience a mix of gratitude for surviving and fear of recurrence. Acknowledging and understanding these emotions is an important step in coping.

2. Physical Recovery: While treatment aims to eliminate cancer, it often leaves survivors dealing with physical changes such as fatigue, pain, or alterations in appearance. Regaining physical strength and addressing any lingering side effects is a gradual process that requires patience and self-care.

3. Psychological Adjustment: The shift from being a patient to a survivor can be challenging. Developing strategies to cope with anxiety, depression, or survivor's guilt is crucial. Professional counseling, therapy, or support groups can provide valuable tools for navigating these emotions.

4. Self-Identity and Relationships: Cancer can reshape how survivors view themselves and how others perceive them. Rebuilding self-esteem, body image, and intimate relationships requires open communication and a supportive network of family and friends.

5. Fear of Recurrence: The fear of cancer returning is a common concern. Survivors can work with healthcare professionals to develop a survivorship care plan that includes regular check-ups, screenings, and a roadmap for managing potential recurrence.

6. Creating a New Routine: As treatment schedules and medical appointments decrease, survivors must establish a new daily routine. This might involve re-entering the workforce, pursuing hobbies, or engaging in activities that bring joy and purpose.

7. Seeking Support: Connecting with fellow survivors and engaging in support groups provides a safe space to share experiences, challenges, and triumphs. Peer support fosters a sense of belonging and helps survivors realize they are not alone in their journey.

8. Mind-Body Well-being: Integrating mindfulness, meditation, and exercise into daily life can promote mental and physical well-being. These practices aid in reducing stress, improving mood, and enhancing overall quality of life.

9. Setting Goals and Moving Forward: Survivorship is an opportunity to set new goals and aspirations. Whether it's pursuing a new career, starting a hobby, or contributing to advocacy efforts, survivors can channel their resilience into positive life changes.

10. Appreciating Life's Moments: After facing a life-threatening illness, survivors often develop a deeper appreciation for life's simple joys. Embracing each day with gratitude and mindfulness can contribute to a more fulfilling post-cancer journey.

8.2 Nurturing Physical and Emotional Well-Being: A Holistic Approach to Health

Achieving a state of well-being encompasses more than just the absence of illness it embraces a balanced synergy between physical and emotional health. In a world marked by constant demands and stressors, prioritizing self-care and adopting holistic practices are essential for nurturing both body and mind.

Physical Well-Being

1. Nutrition: A wholesome diet rich in fruits, vegetables, whole grains, lean proteins, and healthy fats provides the foundation for physical well-being. Nutrient-dense foods fuel the body, boost immunity, and support overall vitality.

2. Exercise: Regular physical activity – whether through cardio, strength training, yoga, or simply walking – promotes cardiovascular health, strengthens muscles, enhances flexibility, and releases endorphins, the "feel-good"hormones.

3. Sleep: Quality sleep is fundamental for rejuvenation and cognitive function. Prioritize a consistent sleep schedule and create a relaxing bedtime routine to ensure restorative rest.

4. Hydration: Drinking an adequate amount of water maintains bodily functions, aids digestion, and helps regulate body temperature. Proper hydration supports healthy skin, organs, and overall vitality.

5. Regular Check-ups: Routine medical check-ups and screenings are crucial for early detection and prevention of potential health issues. Collaborate with healthcare professionals to proactively manage your well-being.

Emotional Well-Being

1. Mindfulness and Meditation: Practicing mindfulness and meditation fosters self-awareness, reduces stress, and enhances emotional resilience. Taking moments to center yourself can lead to greater emotional balance.

2. Positive Relationships: Cultivating meaningful connections and maintaining healthy relationships contribute to emotional well-being. Surround yourself with supportive friends and family who uplift and inspire.

3. Stress Management: Developing effective stress-coping strategies, such as deep breathing, journaling, or engaging in creative activities, helps mitigate the effects of stress and promotes emotional equilibrium.

4. Self-Compassion: Treat yourself with the same kindness and understanding you extend to others. Practice self-compassion by acknowledging your worth, embracing imperfections, and practicing self-care without guilt.

5. Seeking Support: Reach out for professional help when needed. Therapists, counselors, or support groups provide a safe space to discuss emotions, navigate challenges, and develop coping mechanisms.

6. Engaging in Hobbies: Pursuing activities you're passionate about whether it's painting, playing a musical instrument, or gardening fosters a sense of accomplishment, joy, and emotional fulfillment.

Holistic Integration

1. Balancing Act: Strive for a harmonious integration of physical and emotional well-being. Recognize that taking care of your emotional health positively impacts your physical health and vice versa.

2. Self-Reflection: Dedicate time for introspection and self-reflection. Understanding your thoughts, feelings, and behaviors enables you to make informed decisions that support your holistic well-being.

3. Goal Setting: Set realistic goals that encompass both physical and emotional aspects. These goals can range from achieving a fitness milestone to nurturing a positive self-image.

4. Consistency and Patience: Nurturing well-being is an ongoing journey. Consistency and patience are key as you gradually incorporate healthy practices into your daily routine.

8.3 Empowering Unity: Support Groups and Resources for Cancer Survivors

Facing a cancer diagnosis and embarking on the journey of treatment and recovery is an extraordinary feat. Yet, the challenges and emotions that accompany this journey can often feel overwhelming. In these moments, the power of connection and understanding through support groups and resources for cancer survivors becomes invaluable. These platforms serve as beacons of hope, providing a safe haven where survivors can share, learn, and find solace as they navigate the path toward healing and renewed vitality.

The Role of Support Groups

1. Community and Camaraderie: Support groups offer a sense of belonging by bringing together individuals who have experienced similar challenges. Sharing stories, triumphs, and setbacks creates a bond that fosters emotional support and reduces feelings of isolation.

2. Shared Experiences: Survivors can relate to one another on a level that family and friends may not fully understand. The exchange of insights, coping strategies, and advice from those who have walked a similar path can be profoundly comforting.

3. Emotional Healing: Expressing feelings, fears, and hopes within a supportive environment helps survivors process their emotions. This emotional release contributes to a sense of relief and can positively impact mental well-being.

4. Empowerment and Inspiration: Witnessing the strength and resilience of fellow survivors can inspire individuals to overcome challenges, set goals, and take charge of their own recovery.

Resources for Cancer Survivors

1. Online Support Forums: Virtual communities provide a platform for survivors to connect and communicate regardless of geographic location. Online forums facilitate discussions, information sharing, and emotional support.

2. Local Support Groups: In-person support groups organized by hospitals, community centers, or cancer organizations offer a space for survivors to meet face-to-face, share experiences, and access local resources.

3. Counseling and Therapy: Mental health professionals specializing in cancer-related issues offer individual or group therapy sessions to address emotional challenges, anxiety, and stress.

4. Patient Navigators: These dedicated professionals guide survivors through the healthcare system, helping them access resources, understand treatment options, and make informed decisions.

5. Educational Workshops: Workshops and seminars on topics such as nutrition, exercise, survivorship care plans, and managing side effects provide survivors with practical tools for their journey.

6. Art and Expressive Therapies: Creative outlets like art, music, and writing can help survivors process emotions, boost self-esteem, and promote healing.

7. Wellness Retreats: Retreats designed specifically for cancer survivors offer a unique blend of relaxation, emotional healing, and holistic well-being.

Navigating the Path Ahead

1. Finding the Right Fit: Not all support groups or resources are the same. It's important for survivors to explore different options to find a group or resource that aligns with their needs, preferences, and comfort level.

2. Participation and Contribution: Active involvement in support groups allows survivors to not only receive support but also give back by sharing their own experiences and offering encouragement to others.

3. Ongoing Support: The cancer journey is marked by various stages. Survivors may find different groups or resources beneficial at different points, from initial diagnosis to post-treatment survivorship.

Chapter 9

Empowering Health: Strategies for Preventing Cancer Recurrence

Surviving cancer is a remarkable achievement, but the journey doesn't end with remission. Preventing cancer recurrence becomes a paramount goal, inspiring survivors to take proactive steps in maintaining their health and reducing the risk of cancer's return. By adopting a comprehensive approach that combines medical guidance, healthy lifestyle choices, and ongoing vigilance, survivors can navigate the path of prevention with determination and hope.

Medical Follow-Up

1. Regular Check-ups: Consistent medical appointments with oncologists or healthcare professionals are essential. Regular screenings, blood tests, and imaging scans help detect any signs of recurrence at an early stage.

2. Survivorship Care Plan: Collaborate with your medical team to create a tailored survivorship care plan. This plan outlines the recommended follow-up schedule, screenings, and lifestyle recommendations specific to your cancer type and treatment history.

3. Medication Adherence: If prescribed, adhere to medication regimens as directed. Some cancers may require ongoing targeted therapies or hormonal treatments to suppress recurrence.

Healthy Lifestyle Choices

1. Balanced Nutrition: Embrace a diet rich in fruits, vegetables, whole grains, lean proteins, and healthy fats. Limit processed foods, sugary drinks, and red meat while prioritizing foods rich in antioxidants and anti-inflammatory properties.

2. Regular Exercise: Engage in regular physical activity, striving for at least 150 minutes of moderate exercise or 75 minutes of vigorous exercise per week. Exercise supports overall well-being and helps manage weight.

3. Tobacco and Alcohol: Avoid tobacco products and limit alcohol consumption, as these habits are linked to an increased risk of recurrence and other health issues.

4. Maintain a Healthy Weight: Achieving and maintaining a healthy weight reduces the risk of recurrence and improves overall health. A combination of balanced nutrition and regular exercise supports weight management.

5. Stress Management: Incorporate stress-reducing techniques such as mindfulness, meditation, yoga, or deep breathing into your daily routine. Chronic stress can impact the immune system and overall health.

Stay Vigilant

1. Know Your Body: Be attuned to your body's signals and report any unusual symptoms or changes to your healthcare provider promptly. Early detection of potential issues is crucial.

2. Education and Empowerment: Stay informed about your cancer type, treatment, and potential signs of recurrence. Knowledge empowers you to make informed decisions and advocate for your health.

3. Support System: Lean on your support network, whether it's family, friends, or support groups. Sharing your concerns and staying connected can provide emotional strength.

Maintain Positivity and Resilience

1. Mind-Body Connection: Cultivate a positive outlook and emotional resilience. A strong mind-body connection can contribute to improved immune function and overall well-being.

2. Setting Goals: Engage in activities that bring joy, purpose, and fulfillment to your life. Setting and achieving personal goals boosts self-esteem and promotes a sense of accomplishment.

3. Embrace Life: Recognize that each day is an opportunity to embrace life fully. Focus on the present, practice gratitude, and find moments of joy in everyday experiences.

9.1 Navigating Post-Treatment Care and Follow-Up: A Roadmap to Continued Wellness

Completing cancer treatment marks a significant milestone in a survivor's journey, but it also initiates a new phase focused on post-treatment care and follow-up. This stage is essential for monitoring your health, addressing any lingering concerns, and ensuring that you continue to thrive after conquering cancer. By embracing a comprehensive approach that encompasses medical guidance, self-care, and ongoing communication with your healthcare team, you can pave the way for a fulfilling and healthy post-treatment life.

The Importance of Post-Treatment Care

1. Early Detection and Surveillance: Regular medical check-ups, screenings, and tests are essential for detecting any potential signs of recurrence or new health issues at their earliest stages.

2. Managing Late Effects: Some cancer treatments may lead to long-term side effects or health complications. Post-treatment care helps manage and address these effects, enhancing your quality of life.

3. Emotional Well-Being: The emotional aftermath of cancer treatment can be significant. Post-treatment care includes support for managing anxiety, depression, and emotional challenges that may arise.

4. Rebuilding Health: Restoring physical health, strength, and energy levels is a gradual process. Post-treatment care provides guidance for adopting a healthy lifestyle and managing any physical limitations.

Components of Post-Treatment Care

1. Survivorship Care Plan: Collaborate with your medical team to create a personalized survivorship care plan. This plan outlines your treatment history, recommended follow-up schedule, screenings, and ongoing health goals.

2. Medical Follow-Up: Attend scheduled appointments with your oncologist or healthcare provider as outlined in your survivorship care plan. These visits may include physical exams, imaging scans, and blood tests.

3. Screenings: Depending on your cancer type and treatment, you may need regular screenings to monitor for recurrence or new health concerns. Common screenings include mammograms, colonoscopies, and blood tests.

4. Healthy Lifestyle: Adopt a balanced diet, engage in regular exercise, manage stress, and prioritize sleep. These lifestyle choices contribute to your overall well-being and aid in recovery.

5. Managing Side Effects: Report any ongoing or new side effects to your healthcare team. They can provide strategies for managing these effects and improving your comfort.

6. Emotional Support: Seek support from counselors, therapists, or support groups to address emotional challenges and navigate the psychological aspects of post-treatment life.

Navigating Follow-Up Care

1. Open Communication: Maintain open and honest communication with your healthcare team. Share any concerns, symptoms, or changes in your health to ensure timely intervention if needed.

2. Advocate for Yourself: Be an active participant in your post-treatment care. Ask questions, seek clarification, and voice your preferences to ensure your needs are met.

3. Record Keeping: Keep a record of your medical history, treatment details, and test results. This information can aid in discussions with your healthcare team and provide a comprehensive overview of your health.

4. Lifestyle Adjustments: Be patient with yourself as you adapt to life after treatment. Gradually reintegrate into daily activities, listen to your body, and make adjustments as needed.

A Path to Continued Wellness

1. Holistic Approach: Embrace a holistic approach to your well-being, focusing on physical, emotional, and mental health. Nurturing all aspects of your life contributes to a well-rounded and fulfilling post-treatment journey.

2. Advocacy and Empowerment: Take an active role in your health by staying informed, advocating for your needs, and making choices that align with your well-being goals.

3. Celebrating Milestones: Recognize and celebrate your achievements and milestones – both big and small. Each step forward is a testament to your strength and resilience.

9.2 Empowering Long-Term Health: Embracing Lifestyle Modifications

The pursuit of long-term health is a journey that encompasses daily choices and habits, shaping the path toward vitality, well-being, and a fulfilling life. By making intentional lifestyle modifications, individuals can proactively enhance their physical, mental, and emotional health, setting the stage for a vibrant and thriving future. These adjustments, while sometimes requiring effort and commitment, are investments in a life marked by resilience, joy, and the potential for a higher quality of life.

Nutrition

1. Balanced Diet: Embrace a diet rich in whole foods, including a variety of fruits, vegetables, whole grains, lean proteins, and healthy fats. Strive to limit processed foods, sugary snacks, and excessive sodium intake.

2. Portion Control: Be mindful of portion sizes to prevent overeating. Focus on eating until satisfied, not overly full, and choose nutrient-dense options.

3. Hydration: Drink an adequate amount of water daily to support bodily functions, digestion, and overall well-being.

Physical Activity

1. Regular Exercise: Engage in consistent physical activity, combining cardiovascular exercises, strength training, flexibility work, and balance exercises. Aim for at least 150 minutes of moderate exercise or 75 minutes of vigorous exercise each week.

2. Incorporate Movement: Find opportunities to move throughout the day, whether it's taking the stairs, walking during breaks, or practicing yoga. Small, consistent efforts accumulate over time.

Stress Management

1. Mindfulness and Relaxation: Practice mindfulness, deep breathing, meditation, or yoga to manage stress and promote emotional well-being.

2. Hobbies and Creative Outlets: Engage in activities that bring you joy, such as painting, playing a musical instrument, gardening, or writing. These outlets provide a healthy escape from daily stressors.

Sleep

1. Establish a Routine: Create a consistent sleep schedule, aiming for 7-9 hours of quality sleep each night. A calming bedtime routine helps signal your body that it's time to rest.

2. Sleep Environment: Create a comfortable sleep environment by keeping your bedroom dark, quiet, and at a comfortable temperature.

Tobacco and Alcohol

1. Tobacco Avoidance: Refrain from smoking or using tobacco products. Seek resources and support to quit if you are a smoker.

2. Moderate Alcohol Consumption: If you choose to drink alcohol, do so in moderation. For women, this typically means up to one drink per day, and for men, up to two drinks per day.

Social Connections

1. Nurture Relationships: Maintain strong social connections with friends and loved ones. Engage in meaningful conversations and activities that promote a sense of belonging.

2. Support Networks: Participate in support groups, clubs, or organizations that align with your interests and provide opportunities for connection.

Regular Health Screenings

1. Medical Check-ups: Schedule routine medical check-ups and screenings as recommended by healthcare professionals. These screenings detect potential health issues early, when they are most treatable.

2. Dental and Vision Care: Don't overlook oral and eye health. Regular dental cleanings and eye exams contribute to overall well-being.

Positive Mindset

1. Gratitude and Positivity: Cultivate a positive outlook on life by practicing gratitude, focusing on the present moment, and celebrating achievements.

2. Resilience: Develop emotional resilience by adapting to challenges, seeking solutions, and maintaining a growth mindset.

Education and Empowerment

1. Stay Informed: Continuously educate yourself about health, nutrition, and wellness. Knowledge empowers you to make informed choices and take control of your well-being.

2. Self-Advocacy: Advocate for your health by asking questions, seeking second opinions, and actively participating in decisions related to your care.

9.3 Monitoring and Early Detection of Recurrence

Cancer treatment and recovery are significant milestones in a patient's journey, but the threat of recurrence remains a concern. Monitoring and early detection of recurrence play a crucial role in improving patient outcomes and enhancing overall survival rates.

1. Importance of Monitoring: Regular monitoring after cancer treatment is essential to identify any signs of recurrence at the earliest stages. Medical professionals utilize various diagnostic tools, imaging techniques, and laboratory tests to closely track a patient's health status.

2. Surveillance Strategies: Tailored surveillance strategies are designed based on the type of cancer, stage, and individual patient factors. These strategies often involve a combination of physical exams, blood tests (tumor markers), and imaging studies (CT scans, MRIs, PET scans) to detect any abnormal changes in the body.

3. Biomarkers and Liquid Biopsies: Emerging technologies like liquid biopsies are transforming the landscape of recurrence monitoring. These tests analyze circulating tumor DNA (ctDNA) and other biomarkers in the blood, providing a non-invasive method to detect early signs of cancer recurrence.

4. Patient Engagement: Patients are encouraged to actively participate in their post-treatment journey by reporting any unusual symptoms, changes, or discomfort to their healthcare team. Open communication between patients and medical professionals is vital for effective monitoring.

5. Advances in Imaging: Cutting-edge imaging techniques, such as functional MRI and positron emission tomography (PET), offer detailed insights into cellular activity and metabolism. These advanced methods aid in detecting tiny abnormalities that might indicate recurrence.

6. Artificial Intelligence (AI) and Machine Learning: AI-powered algorithms analyze vast amounts of patient data to identify subtle patterns and anomalies that may go unnoticed by traditional methods. These technologies enhance the accuracy of recurrence detection.

7. Psychosocial Support: Coping with the fear of recurrence is an integral part of a patient's emotional well-being. Support groups, counseling, and survivorship programs offer psychological support, helping patients manage anxiety and stress.

8. Early Intervention: Detecting recurrence at an early stage allows for prompt intervention, which can include targeted therapies, surgical options, or radiation treatments. Early detection significantly improves the chances of successful treatment.

9. Multidisciplinary Approach: A collaborative approach involving oncologists, radiologists, pathologists, and other specialists ensures a comprehensive assessment of a patient's health status, increasing the likelihood of timely recurrence detection.

10. Future Outlook: Research continues to refine monitoring techniques, making them more sensitive and accurate. The integration of genomics, proteomics, and other 'omics' technologies holds promise for even more precise and personalized recurrence monitoring.

Chapter 10

Empowering Yourself and Loved Ones

Empowerment is a transformative journey that involves gaining confidence, knowledge, and the ability to take control of one's life. When you empower yourself, you not only enhance your own well-being but also inspire and uplift those around you, including your loved ones. Here are some key aspects of empowering yourself and your loved ones:

1. Self-Awareness and Reflection: Empowerment begins with self-awareness. Take time to reflect on your strengths, weaknesses, goals, and values. Understand your emotions, triggers, and aspirations. This self-awareness serves as a foundation for personal growth and positive change.

2. Education and Learning: Knowledge is a powerful tool for empowerment. Continuously seek opportunities to learn and expand your skills. Whether it's pursuing higher education, attending workshops, or simply reading books, acquiring knowledge opens doors to new possibilities.

3. Setting Boundaries: Empowerment involves setting healthy boundaries in various aspects of life. Clearly define your limits and communicate them assertively. This practice fosters self-respect and helps prevent situations that could lead to stress or discomfort.

4. Effective Communication: Enhance your communication skills to express your thoughts, needs, and feelings effectively. Open and honest communication strengthens relationships and promotes understanding among loved ones.

5. Building Resilience: Empowerment equips you with the resilience needed to navigate challenges. Develop coping strategies, practice mindfulness, and cultivate a positive mindset. Resilience enables you to bounce back from setbacks and maintain emotional well-being.

6. Goal Setting and Action: Empowerment is about taking purposeful action toward your goals. Set realistic and achievable objectives, and create a plan to work toward them. Each step you take reinforces your sense of empowerment.

7. Support Networks: Surround yourself with a supportive network of friends, family, and mentors who uplift and encourage you. These connections provide emotional support and guidance along your empowerment journey.

8. Encouraging Loved Ones: Empowerment is contagious. By empowering yourself, you inspire and motivate your loved ones to do the same. Encourage their dreams, provide a listening ear, and offer guidance when needed.

9. Respecting Diversity: Recognize and celebrate the diversity of perspectives and experiences within your family and social circles. Empowerment involves respecting and valuing the uniqueness of each individual.

10. Giving Back: Empowerment is not only about personal growth but also about making a positive impact on others and the community. Engage in acts of kindness, volunteer work, or mentorship to empower others to reach their potential.

11. Mind-Body Connection: Empowerment extends to taking care of your physical and mental health. Prioritize self-care through regular exercise, balanced nutrition, relaxation techniques, and seeking professional support when needed.

12. Embracing Change: Empowerment involves embracing change as an opportunity for growth. Embrace new experiences, adapt to challenges, and view change as a chance to evolve and improve.

10.1 Advocating for Your Health: Communicating with Medical Professionals

Effective communication with medical professionals is a cornerstone of proactive healthcare and a key component of advocating for your well-being. When you actively engage in conversations with your healthcare team, you contribute to better decision-making, accurate diagnoses, and personalized treatment plans. Here's how to advocate for your health through clear and open communication:

1. Prepare and Organize: Before appointments, make a list of your symptoms, concerns, and questions. Prioritize the most important ones to ensure you address all relevant issues during your visit.

2. Active Listening: Listen carefully to your healthcare provider's explanations, recommendations, and instructions. Ask for clarification if something is unclear and take notes to remember important details.

3. Be Honest and Open: Share your complete medical history, including any pre-existing conditions, medications, allergies, and lifestyle factors. Honesty enables your medical team to make well-informed decisions.

4. Ask Questions: Don't hesitate to ask questions about your condition, tests, treatment options, and potential side effects. Understanding your situation empowers you to make informed choices.

5. Clarify Terminology: If you don't understand medical jargon, ask your healthcare provider to explain concepts in simpler terms. Clear explanations promote better comprehension.

6. Express Your Concerns: If you have reservations about a particular treatment or procedure, voice your concerns. A collaborative approach allows you and your healthcare provider to explore alternatives.

7. Discuss Goals: Clearly state your health goals and preferences. Whether it's pain management, maintaining functionality, or pursuing certain treatments, aligning your goals with your medical team helps guide decision-making.

8. Share Changes: If your condition changes or worsens between appointments, notify your healthcare provider promptly. Timely updates enable adjustments to your care plan.

9. Explore Options: In situations where treatment choices are available, discuss the pros and cons of each option. Work with your medical team to choose what aligns best with your values and priorities.

10. Involve Loved Ones: If appropriate, bring a trusted family member or friend to appointments. They can provide support, help you remember details, and ask questions you might overlook.

11. Request Second Opinions: If you're uncertain about a diagnosis or treatment plan, seeking a second opinion can offer valuable insights and reassurance.

12. Follow-Up: After appointments, review your notes and follow any instructions provided by your medical team. If you have concerns or questions, don't hesitate to reach out.

13. Respectful Communication: Maintain a respectful and collaborative attitude when discussing your health. Effective communication promotes a positive relationship with your medical professionals.

14. Utilize Online Resources: Trusted medical websites and resources can provide additional information and support your understanding of your condition and treatment options.

15. Advocacy Organizations: Depending on your health condition, there may be advocacy organizations that offer information, resources, and a community of individuals with similar experiences.

10.2 Educating Family and Friends about Cancer Prevention

Cancer prevention is a shared responsibility that involves making informed lifestyle choices and adopting healthy habits. By educating your family and friends about cancer prevention, you empower them to take proactive steps toward reducing their risk of developing this complex disease. Here's how to effectively educate your loved ones about cancer prevention:

1. Start Conversations: Initiate open and non-judgmental discussions about cancer prevention. Create a comfortable environment where questions and concerns can be freely addressed.

2. Share Reliable Information: Provide accurate and evidence-based information about cancer risk factors, such as tobacco use, unhealthy diet, lack of physical activity, exposure to UV radiation, and more.

3. Use Clear Language: Use simple and relatable language when explaining complex medical concepts. Avoid jargon that might confuse or discourage understanding.

4. Highlight Benefits of Prevention: Emphasize the positive impact of cancer prevention, such as improved overall health, increased energy levels, and a reduced risk of chronic diseases beyond cancer.

5. Provide Resources: Share brochures, articles, videos, and online resources from reputable sources like cancer research institutions and health organizations.

6. Host Educational Events: Organize workshops, seminars, or virtual sessions where experts can discuss cancer prevention strategies, debunk myths, and answer questions.

7. Encourage Regular Check-Ups: Stress the importance of regular health check-ups and screenings for early detection of cancer or precancerous conditions.

8. Promote Healthy Lifestyle Habits: Educate your loved ones about the significance of maintaining a balanced diet, staying physically active, avoiding tobacco and excessive alcohol consumption, and protecting skin from UV radiation.

9. Lead by Example: Adopt healthy habits yourself to serve as a role model for your family and friends. Your actions can inspire others to make positive changes.

10. Customize Recommendations: Recognize that different individuals have different risk factors. Tailor your education to their specific needs and circumstances.

11. Address Myths and Misconceptions: Correct any misconceptions or myths about cancer that might be prevalent among your family and friends. Use factual information to dispel false beliefs.

12. Use Personal Stories: Share stories of individuals who successfully made lifestyle changes to reduce their cancer risk. Personal narratives can be impactful and relatable.

13. Engage Social Media: Utilize social media platforms to share informative posts, articles, infographics, and videos on cancer prevention.

14. Encourage Supportive Networks: Encourage your loved ones to support and motivate each other in adopting healthy behaviors. Group efforts can make prevention more enjoyable and effective.

15. Celebrate Achievements: Celebrate milestones and successes in adopting healthier lifestyles. Positive reinforcement reinforces the importance of ongoing efforts.

16. Stay Updated: Continue educating yourself about the latest advancements in cancer prevention. Share new insights and findings with your family and friends.

10.3 Inspiring Hope and Encouragement in the Face of Cancer

Cancer, a word that carries a weight beyond its letters, is a battle that millions of individuals around the world confront. While the journey may seem daunting, it's essential to remember that hope and encouragement can serve as powerful allies, guiding those affected by cancer towards brighter days. In this article, we delve into the transformative role of hope and encouragement in the face of cancer, highlighting stories of resilience, support systems, and strategies for nurturing a positive mindset.

The Power of Hope:
Hope is the beacon that shines through the darkest of times. When grappling with a cancer diagnosis, hope

becomes an anchor that keeps individuals grounded and determined. It's the belief that a better outcome is possible, no matter how challenging the circumstances. Hope inspires individuals to embrace their treatment journey with an unwavering spirit, focusing on progress and the potential for healing. From groundbreaking medical advancements to stories of survivors who defied the odds, hope fuels the fire of determination and keeps the light of possibility burning.

Building a Supportive Network:
Encouragement often arrives in the form of a helping hand, a listening ear, or a heartfelt message. Cancer's impact is not limited to the individual diagnosed; it reverberates through families, friends, and communities. Creating a robust support network plays a pivotal role in sustaining hope and providing strength. Loved ones offer companionship, empathy, and a safe space to share fears and triumphs. Support groups, both in-person and online, serve as spaces where experiences are exchanged, bonds are formed, and the power of collective encouragement is harnessed.

Cultivating Resilience:
Resilience is the art of bouncing back stronger, even in the face of adversity. Cancer challenges individuals to tap into their inner well of resilience, discovering newfound depths of strength they may not have known existed. The journey may be arduous, but with each step, resilience grows. Embracing mindfulness, practicing self-compassion, and engaging in activities that bring joy contribute to cultivating resilience. By acknowledging challenges while focusing on personal growth, individuals can emerge from the cancer journey transformed and fortified.

Harnessing Positive Mindset:
The mind wields incredible influence over our
well-being. Cultivating a positive mindset is a vital
aspect of the cancer journey, as it shapes how one
perceives and navigates challenges. Visualization
techniques, meditation, and gratitude exercises
empower individuals to reframe their perspective and
focus on the silver linings. Celebrating small victories,
nurturing a sense of humor, and embracing creativity
can infuse each day with positivity, serving as a source
of strength and encouragement.

Celebrating Milestones:
In the battle against cancer, every milestone achieved
deserves celebration. Whether it's completing a round of
treatment, reaching a remission milestone, or simply
experiencing a day of improved well-being,
acknowledging these victories is a way of honoring
progress and finding encouragement. These milestones
symbolize the determination, resilience, and hope that
drive individuals forward, inspiring them to continue
fighting and embracing life's precious moments.

Chapter 11

Embracing a Proactive Approach to Cancer Control and Combat

In the ongoing battle against cancer, the significance of a proactive approach cannot be overstated. As the prevalence of cancer continues to rise globally, it becomes increasingly imperative to shift our focus from reactive treatments to proactive measures that encompass prevention, early detection, and comprehensive combat strategies. Embracing this proactive approach holds the potential to revolutionize the way we perceive and address cancer, leading to improved patient outcomes, reduced healthcare burdens, and a brighter future for all.

1. Prevention as the First Line of Defense

Preventing cancer is undeniably more effective and cost-efficient than treating it. By promoting healthier lifestyles, such as adopting balanced diets, engaging in regular physical activity, avoiding tobacco and excessive alcohol consumption, and protecting oneself from harmful environmental factors, individuals can significantly reduce their risk of developing certain types of cancer. Community education, public awareness campaigns, and policy initiatives play pivotal roles in encouraging these lifestyle changes on a broader scale.

2. Early Detection for Enhanced Survival Rates

Early detection remains a critical factor in successful cancer treatment. Regular screenings, self-examinations, and advanced diagnostic technologies can identify cancer at its nascent stages, enabling medical professionals to initiate timely interventions. Efforts to ensure accessibility to screenings and to raise awareness about the importance of early detection are essential components of a proactive strategy.

3. Tailored Treatment Approaches

Advancements in cancer research have led to the development of personalized treatment approaches. Precision medicine, which tailors therapies based on an individual's genetic makeup and specific cancer characteristics, enhances treatment efficacy while minimizing adverse effects. Embracing these innovations and integrating them into standard healthcare practices amplifies the proactive nature of cancer combat.

4. Collaborative Efforts and Research
Proactive cancer control requires collaborative efforts among researchers, healthcare providers, policymakers, and the community. Investments in research to uncover novel prevention methods, diagnostic tools, and treatment modalities are pivotal in shaping the landscape of cancer care. Additionally, fostering multidisciplinary collaborations enables the exchange of knowledge and the formulation of comprehensive strategies.

5. Empowerment Through Education

Educating individuals about cancer risks, prevention strategies, and the importance of early detection empowers them to take charge of their health. Through informative campaigns, workshops, and educational resources, people can make informed decisions and actively participate in their own well-being.

Embracing a proactive approach to cancer control and combat requires a collective commitment to change. By promoting prevention, early detection, tailored treatments, collaboration, and education, we pave the way for a future where the impact of cancer is significantly reduced. As medical science evolves and our understanding of cancer deepens, embracing a proactive stance holds the promise of transforming the lives of countless individuals and families, offering them hope and the potential for a healthier and brighter tomorrow.

11.1 The Journey Towards a Cancer-Free Future

Cancer, a formidable adversary that has affected countless lives worldwide, continues to inspire relentless efforts towards a future free from its grasp. This journey, marked by scientific breakthroughs, tireless advocacy, and unwavering determination, embodies the collective commitment of researchers, healthcare professionals, survivors, caregivers, and communities alike. As we traverse this path towards a cancer-free future, each stride brings us closer to the realization of a world where cancer's impact is significantly diminished.

1. Research and Innovation

The cornerstone of our journey lies in the realm of research and innovation. Scientists and medical experts delve into the intricate mechanisms of cancer, striving to unravel its complexities and uncover novel treatment strategies. From targeted therapies and immunotherapies to advances in early detection technologies, every breakthrough is a step forward in the battle against cancer's relentless advance.

2. Empowerment through Awareness

Empowering individuals with knowledge about cancer's risks, prevention, and early detection is a pivotal aspect of our journey. Awareness campaigns and educational initiatives equip people with the tools they need to make informed decisions about their health. By understanding the importance of regular screenings, adopting healthier lifestyles, and recognizing potential symptoms, individuals become active participants in their own well-being.

3. Patient-Centered Care

At the heart of our journey are those who have faced cancer firsthand, the patients and their families. Patient-centered care focuses on providing holistic support, tailored treatments, and compassionate guidance throughout the cancer experience. This approach recognizes that each person's journey is unique and seeks to enhance their quality of life as they navigate the challenges of diagnosis, treatment, and recovery.

4. Collaborative Networks

Collaboration forms a crucial thread in the fabric of our journey. Researchers, medical institutions, nonprofits, government agencies, and philanthropic organizations come together to pool their expertise, resources, and insights. Through these partnerships, we amplify our collective impact, accelerate progress, and drive positive change in the fight against cancer.

5. Survivorship and Resilience

Survivors and their stories inspire hope and resilience, serving as beacons of light along the journey. Their experiences demonstrate the power of the human spirit to overcome adversity and thrive in the face of challenges. By sharing their journeys, survivors foster a sense of community and solidarity that empowers others to navigate their own paths with courage and determination.

6. Advocacy and Policy

Advocates play a pivotal role in shaping the landscape of cancer care. By raising awareness, championing research funding, and advocating for policies that prioritize cancer prevention and treatment, they catalyze change on both local and global levels. Their voices amplify the urgency of the journey towards a cancer-free future.

As we journey towards a cancer-free future, each milestone achieved is a testament to the unwavering dedication of countless individuals who refuse to accept the status quo. While challenges persist, the indomitable human spirit and the relentless pursuit of scientific knowledge fuel our progress.

The road ahead may be arduous, but with every stride we take, we inch closer to a world where cancer is no longer a formidable foe, but a conquerable challenge.

Together, we hold the power to shape this future, a future defined by resilience, compassion, and the triumph of the human spirit over one of the most formidable adversaries of our time.